MCQs in Sports Medicine

MCQs in Sports Medicine

Conor O'Brien
MB LRCPSI MSc DSMLU DSMRSC DSMSA DMSKEL ABSM CSCN EMG FACSM

Lecturer in Sports Medicine at the Royal College of Surgeons in Ireland,
Consultant Clinical Neurophysiologist and Physician in Physical and Sports Medicine at Dublin's Blackrock Clinic

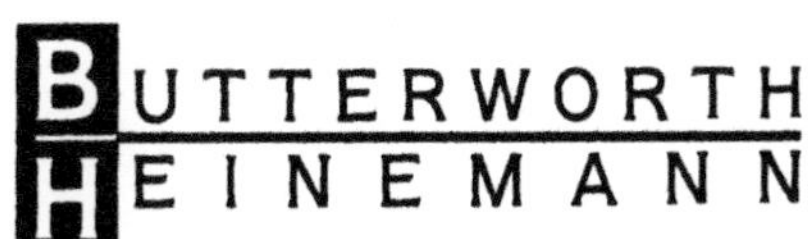

OXFORD AUCKLAND BOSTON JOHANNESBURG MELBOURNE NEW DELHI

Butterworth-Heinemann
Linacre House, Jordan Hill, Oxford OX2 8DP
225 Wildwood Avenue, Woburn, MA 01801-2041
A division of Reed Educational and Professional Publishing Ltd

A member of the Reed Elsevier plc group

First published 1999

British Library Cataloguing in Publication Data
A catalogue record for this book is available from the British Library

Library of Congress Cataloguing in Publication Data
A catalogue record for this book is available from the Library of Congress

ISBN 0 7506 2949 5

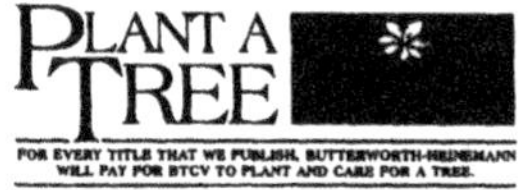

Transferred to digital printing 2006.

Contents

Introduction

This book is designed as a primer in sports medicine for postgraduate doctors whose practice encompasses the treatment and preparation of both elite and recreational athletes, and the counselling of individuals who wish to improve their overall health by an exercise intervention programme. It is not meant to be a definitive text, but rather a practical approach to the assessment of knowledge relating to commonly encountered problems in the practice of sports medicine.

How to use this book

For each question a condition or situation is presented, followed by a list of statements which are either true or false. You should work through these statements, and through each question within a section. With the answers you will find a short review of the topic, which includes information referring to each statement and a reference for further reading.

These references will, in the author's opinion, give the reader a particular insight into the subject and a more rounded approach to it.

The topics covered in this text are those that will regularly be seen in clinical sports medicine outpatient clinics, and may present to primary care, rheumatological or orthopaedic services.

It is hoped that this book will be of value to the postgraduate doctor who is training and preparing for sports medicine certification, and to those in practice with an interest in this expanding specialty.

About the author

Conor O'Brien is a graduate of the Royal College of Surgeons in Ireland. He completed his internal medicine training in Dublin before embarking on a career in sports medicine and neurophysiology.

He initially studied at the Royal London Hospital in the Department of Sports Medicine, where he gained a Diploma and a Masters degree in Sports Medicine, and the Diploma of the Royal Scottish Colleges and Apothecaries of London. He subsequently worked in North America, where he was certified by the American Boards of Sports Medicine. He is a Fellow of the American College of Sports Medicine. Dr O'Brien subsequently trained in clinical neurophysiology at the University of Washington, Seattle, before returning to his native Ireland, where he is in practice as a consultant clinical neurophysiologist and sports medicine physician. He is Lecturer in Sports Medicine at the Royal College of Surgeons in Ireland, has a clinical attachment to the Irish National Maternity Hospital as a consultant neurophysiologist, and is in private practice in Dublin's Blackrock Clinic.

Dr O'Brien's own sporting interests include rugby and golf. He was team physician to the Irish Olympic team at the Centennial games in Atlanta, and has travelled with the senior Leinster rugby union squad as team doctor. His research interests include substance abuse among the athletic population, exercise prescription and sports-related neuropathy assessment.

He is married to Aine, a general practitioner; they have three daughters, Laura-Enya, Aoife and Sorcha, and live in Dublin.

Part I Questions

General medicine

1. **Cluster headaches:**
   a. Cluster headaches usually last 6 hours or more.
   b. They cause nausea and vomiting.
   c. They commonly cause stabbing pain around the eye.
   d. They always have a prodromal phase.
   e. They preclude participation in contact sports.

2. **Herpes simplex skin infections:**
   a. Skin infections are successfully treated with acyclovir in the vesicular phase.
   b. They can be caused by the stress of competition.
   c. Equipment hygiene will not affect spread.
   d. They can cause salpingitis.
   e. They rarely occur in wrestlers, due to the use of head guards.

3. **Sudden death in athletes:**
   a. Idiopathic concentric left ventricular hypertrophy is found in 10–18 per cent of cases of sudden cardiac death in athletes.
   b. Sudden death is defined as death within 48 hours of the onset of symptoms.
   c. The aetiology of sudden death varies with respect to age.
   d. Cardiac arrhythmia is the most common cause of sudden death in athletes over 35 years of age.
   e. Congenital cardiac abnormalities are the predominant cause of sudden death in younger athletes.

4. **Exercise-induced asthma:**
   a. This affects less than 1 per cent of the general population.
   b. Air pollutants do not affect EIA.
   c. EIA is made worse by exercising in a humid environment.
   d. EIA occurs most often 6–8 minutes into a programme at moderate to high intensities of exercise.
   e. Most individuals with EIA take regular exercise.

5. **Athletic anaemia:**
   a. Oral iron may be of haematological and physiological benefit in the non-anaemic state.
   b. The physiological anaemia often observed in endurance athletes is similar to the anaemia of pregnancy.
   c. The pseudo-anaemia observed in athletes probably arises from a significantly expanded plasma volume and a decrease in red cell mass.
   d. There is increased red cell destruction during exercise.
   e. Oral iron should routinely be recommended for the exercising athlete.

6. **Temperature and exercise:**
   a. Core temperature increases during dynamic exercise.
   b. Changes in core temperature are dependent on ambient temperature.
   c. The skin surface temperature falls during the initial stages of exercise.
   d. Surface skin temperature changes are related to thermal factors such as skin sweating.
   e. The surface mechanism fails when the core body temperature falls below 34°C.

7. **Lipids and exercise:**
   a. Elevated HDL2 is positively associated with the development of coronary artery disease.
   b. Apoprotein B is considered to be protective against coronary artery disease.
   c. Dietary fibre does not affect the lipoprotein profile.
   d. HDL, HDL2 and apoprotein A1 levels are elevated following alcohol intake.
   e. Apoprotein A1 is the major protein in HDL.

8. **Dehydration:**
    a. Dehydration of 2–3 per cent of the body weight can significantly affect aerobic performance.
    b. Dehydration does not significantly impair thermal regulation.
    c. Dehydration can decrease the blood volume but does not affect blood pressure.
    d. A weight loss of 1 kg indicates that the athlete requires to rehydrate by 2 l of fluid, using the daily weight method of hydration assessment.
    e. Over 60 per cent of our daily water intake is obtained from the food we eat, and approximately 30 per cent from our daily water intake. The remaining 10 per cent is produced in our cells during metabolism.

9. **Exercise-induced asthma: The following are high-risk sports for individuals susceptible to exercise-induced asthma:**
    a. Soccer.
    b. Tennis.
    c. Gymnastics.
    d. Basketball.
    e. Rowing.

10. **Management of exercise-induced asthma:**
    a. The incidence of exercise-induced asthma in the general population is between 10 and 15 per cent.
    b. FEV1 and FEV1-FEC values below 80 per cent of predicted values are better indicators of obstructive airways disease than peak flow measurements.
    c. Inhaled corticosteroids, if used regularly, can enhance the effectiveness of beta agonists.
    d. Inhaled corticosteroids act as an effective bronchodilator.
    e. Inhaled doses of corticosteroids of 400 gm daily have a high incidence of side effects.

11. **Herpes virus infections:**
    a. Human herpes virus-8 is the herpes strain associated with herpes gladiatorium.
    b. Human herpes virus-6 is suggested to be an aetiological factor in multiple sclerosis.
    c. Herpes virus type 1 can cause a development of erythema multiforme.
    d. Acyclovir is specific for herpes viruses, as the phosphorylation required for its activation occurs only in cells infected with herpes.
    e. Prompt treatment at the prodromal phase of herpes type 1 viral infection may abort an attack, but antiviral treatment has only a modest effect if begun after the vesicles have formed.

12. **Exercise-induced anaphylaxis: This is associated with the following:**
    a. Pruritus.
    b. Syncope.
    c. Blurred vision.
    d. Temporal headache.
    e. Small weals of less than 4 mm on the skin surface.

13. **Sickle-cell trait and sudden death:**
    a. The risk of sudden death in athletes with sickle-cell trait is approximately 1 in 100 000 for the 20–30 years age group.
    b. Reduction of the risk of exertional collapse associated with sickle-cell trait is achieved by use of antihistamines.
    c. The black African community has a significantly increased risk of this disorder.
    d. Training at altitudes of 3000 m (~10 000 ft) is associated with increase risk of exertional collapse in individuals with sickle-cell trait.
    e. Death is caused by vascular occlusion and intravascular coagulation.

14. **Peripheral arterial disease:**
    a. Peripheral arterial disease affects 12 per cent of the general population.
    b. Cessation of smoking appears to improve claudication symptoms in individuals with peripheral arterial disease.
    c. Improvement in the hypertension status does not improve claudication symptoms in these cases.
    d. Walking exercise training is associated with improvement in treadmill exercise performance in these individuals.
    e. Walking exercise training is associated with improvement in symptoms of exercise-related claudication.

15. **Hamstrings:**
    a. The semimembranosus hamstring receives its nerve supply from the peroneal portion of the sciatic nerve.
    b. The short head of the biceps femoris receives its nerve supply from the tibial portion of the sciatic nerve.
    c. The long head of the biceps femoris muscle receives its nerve supply from the peroneal portion of the sciatic nerve.
    d. The long and short head of the biceps femoris muscles receives its predominant root supply from the level of L4–5.
    e. The semimembranosus receives its predominant nerve root supply from the S1, S2 lumbar root levels.
    f. The biceps femoris is inserted below the knee as the pes anserina.
    g. The semimembranosus and semitendinosus are the internal or medial hamstrings.

16. **Altitude sickness:**
    a. Altitude sickness occurs within 30 minutes of ascent.
    b. Acute altitude sickness is associated with insomnia.
    c. High altitude pulmonary oedema (HAPO) is a life-threatening condition requiring acute emergency management.
    d. HAPO becomes more prevalent as the climber ages.
    e. High altitude cerebral oedema (HACO) usually occurs at a level of 3 000 metres.

The team physician

17. **Acute management of a quadriceps haematoma: Appropriate treatment would include the following:**
    a. Ice.
    b. Compression.
    c. Elevation.
    d. Non-steroidal agents.
    e. Ultrasound.

18. **Delayed onset muscle soreness:**
    a. Delayed onset muscle soreness (DOMS) occurs within 24–48 hours of exercise.
    b. DOMS is associated with elevated plasma muscle enzymes.
    c. DOMS is associated with myoglobinuria.
    d. Higher levels of DOMS is associated with concentric rather than eccentric activity.
    e. DOMS may be associated with structural damage to the contractile filament.

19. **The female athletic triad:**
    a. The female athlete triad involves three conditions: bulimia, amenorrhoea and osteoporosis.
    b. The female athlete triad consists of three conditions: eating disorder, amenorrhoea and hirsutism.
    c. Disordered eating patterns are similar in young female athletes and dancers.
    d. The female athletic triad is a self-limiting condition.
    e. All female athletes who present with stress fractures or menstrual irregularities should be screened for the female athletic triad.

20. **Spondylolisthesis:**
    a. An adolescent with spondylolisthesis of 50 per cent or more should not participate in vigorous sport.
    b. The defect in spondylolisthesis occurs at the spinous process.
    c. Spondylolisthesis prohibits the patient undergoing isokinetic dynamometry.
    d. The spondylitic defect is always visible on plain radiographs.
    e. Spondylolisthesis is always traumatic.

21. **Whiplash injury:**
    a. Neck pain is the commonest symptom encountered after a whiplash injury.
    b. Neck pain is an immediate symptom in a true cantilever whiplash injury.
    c. Headache is seen in over 50 per cent of patients presenting with whiplash injury.
    d. There is an increased incidence of degenerative change at the C5/6/7 level at long-term follow-up following a whiplash injury.
    e. Individuals with a true whiplash injury will be pain-free after 2 years.

22. **Exertional compartment syndrome of the leg:**
    a. The anterior and deep posterior compartments are the most commonly involved.
    b. The lateral and deep posterior compartments are the most commonly involved.
    c. The tibial nerve runs through the lateral compartment, and may be compromised by a lateral compartment syndrome.
    d. Acute exertional compartment syndrome is most commonly seen in professional athletes.
    e. Chronic compartment syndrome is associated with activity-related pain beginning at a predictable time after starting exercise.

23. **Emotional stress:**
    a. Pre-competition heart rates are not significantly elevated in American football players.
    b. Soccer players and motor racing drivers have significantly elevated pre-competition heart rates.
    c. Higher levels of anxiety among footballers are associated with lower injury rates due to a heightened reaction state.
    d. Stress hormones are elevated most in those playing positions with the greatest responsibility.
    e. Increased stress caused by competitive sport can lead to enlargement of the thyroid gland.

24. **Swimmer's shoulder:**
    a. Swimmer's shoulder is usually caused by subacromial impingement syndrome.
    b. It is most common with freestyle swimmers and breaststrokers.
    c. It can affect up to 75 per cent of all competitive swimmers.
    d. Nerve conduction of the axillary nerve function is an essential component of the work up.
    e. Impingement can occur during the early and mid pull-through phase of the freestyle stroke.

25. **Wet bulb temperature:**
    a. The wet bulb temperature (WBT) never exceeds the dry bulb temperature.
    b. Wet bulb temperature readings greater than 25°C suggest that exercise should be postponed.
    c. The wet bulb globe temperature index can readily identify conditions of heat stress.
    d. The wet bulb globe temperature index is a function of the dry bulb temperature, the wet bulb temperature and the globe temperature.
    e. When the wet bulb temperature equals the dry bulb temperature, the air is completely saturated with water vapour and there is a relative humidity equal to 100 per cent.

26. **Nasal injury**:
    a. Epistaxis originating from the Kiesselbach's area is usually controlled by pinching the nose for 2–5 minutes.
    b. Posterior epistaxis may need positioning and packing if local pressure fails to arrest the bleeding.
    c. Cartilage injuries may occur in association with septal haematomas.
    d. Profuse epistaxis following fracture is generally from the anterior ethmoidal artery.
    e. Nasal lacerations causing cartilage injury are best left untreated.

27. **Elbow pain in the tennis-playing population:**
    a. Fifty per cent of elbow pain is localized to the lateral epicondyle at the attachment of the common extensor muscles.
    b. Twenty-five per cent of elbow pain is at the medial epicondyle attachment of the flexor origin.
    c. Eight per cent of elbow pain in tennis players is posterior, around the olecranon process.
    d. Over 90 per cent of elbow pain related to tennis playing effects the lateral structures only.
    e. Anterior interosseous nerve entrapment is a rare cause of lateral elbow pain among the tennis playing population.

28. **Sports brassieres:**
    a. Women with a B cup size or smaller should use an encapsulating bra during exercise.
    b. Women with C cup size or greater should use a compressive bra when participating in sport.
    c. Bra straps should be wide and elasticated.
    d. The fabric should be at least 50 per cent cotton.
    e. Seams should intersect the nipple line.

29. **Biomechanical abnormalities:**
    a. Femoral anteversion is a frequent cause of the patellofemoral syndrome.
    b. Genu varum is a frequent cause of the patellofemoral syndrome.
    c. Genu valgum is a common cause of the ilio-tibial band friction syndrome.
    d. Pes planus is a frequent predisposing factor to patellofemoral syndrome.
    e. Pes cavus may predispose the athlete to Achilles tendonitis.

30. **Tineanea cruris:**
    a. Tineanea cruris is a frequent complaint among elite female athletes.
    b. The incidence is decreased by wearing athletic supports.
    c. Athletic apparel made from synthetic materials reduces the incidence.
    d. It is most common in athletes with heavily muscled thighs.
    e. Acyclovir is the treatment of choice.

31. **Rhabdomyolysis:**
    a. Rhabdomyolysis can be cause by an air embolism.
    b. It can be caused by intensive exercise.
    c. This can be caused by a hornet's sting.
    d. Rhabdomyolysis is commonly associated with exercise.
    e. It is associated with acute renal failure.

32. **Injuries to the male genito-urinary system:**
    a. Sexually transmitted diseases are common urological problems in athletes.
    b. 'Bicycler's Penis' is paraesthesia and numbness in the perineum and phallus that is associated with prolonged bicycle riding.
    c. Most genito-urinary system injuries result from a direct blow, and require prompt evaluation.
    d. A testicular mass separate from the cord and epididymis implies a varicocele and does not require any further investigation.
    e. Varicoceles can be present in up to 19 per cent of all men.

33. **Heat cramps:**
    a. Heat cramps usually occur in the calf muscle after exercise.
    b. Heat cramps may occur in association with hypernatraemia.
    c. Heat cramps are associated with a core temperature greater than 39°C.
    d. Heat cramps may mimic an acute appendix.
    e. Heat cramps usually remit spontaneously, and the athlete is safe to return to activity after half an hour's rest.

34. **Osgood–Schlatter's disease:**
    a. In Osgood–Schlatter's disease, there can be patellar tendon thickening.
    b. There may be obliteration of the inferior angle of the infrapatellar fat pad.
    c. There may be fragmentation of the tibial tuberosity.
    d. Fragmentation of the tibial tuberosity is the most commonly encountered X-ray finding.
    e. Radiological changes are best observed on lateral X-rays, with the tibia in slight external rotation.

35. **Sinding-Larsen–Johansson disease:**
    a. Sinding-Larsen–Johansson (SLJ) disease commonly affects the 8–10-year-old population.
    b. It is exacerbated by kneeling.
    c. Radiological calcification is always observed.
    d. SLJ disease usually requires surgical intervention.
    e. Calcification of the inferior pole can often yield a normal appearance in chronic cases.

36. **Tietze's syndrome:**
    a. Tietze's syndrome usually affects the second and third costochondral junctions.
    b. It always has a traumatic origin.
    c. It rarely affects young females.
    d. It is associated with respiratory tract infections.
    e. It is associated with fibrositis syndrome.

Sports injuries

37. **Iliac crest apophysitis:**
    a. Iliac crest apophysitis is an overuse injury commonly seen in horse riders.
    b. Ober's test is positive in ilio-tibial band syndrome and iliac crest apophysitis.
    c. There is usually a history of trauma.
    d. It is most common in the adolescent growth spurt.
    e. X-rays can be normal.

38. **Posterior interosseous neuropathy:**
    a. The posterior interosseous nerve (PIN) is a branch of the radial nerve.
    b. The posterior interosseous nerve can be entrapped by the pronator teres muscle.
    c. PIN syndrome is associated with EMG abnormalities in the extensor indices muscle.
    d. PIN syndrome may mimic a medial epicondylitis injury.
    e. PIN syndrome can cause a loss of sensation in the ring and little fingers.

39. **Lower limb athletic neuropathy:**
    a. Meralgia paraesthetica can occur in weight-lifters due to tight belts and trusses.
    b. The saphenous nerve can be compressed in the lateral aspects of the knee, and this is seen in surfers.
    c. Piriformis syndrome is a common cause of sciatica in the athlete.
    d. Sural neuropathy can be caused by trauma from ski boots.
    e. Peroneal neuropathy is rarely encountered in sportsmen and women.

40. **Ulnar collateral ligament injury (skier's thumb):**
    a. This is usually caused by a forced abduction injury to the thumb.
    b. The key pinch grip becomes weak.
    c. A Sterner lesion always requires surgical repair.
    d. Stressing the thumb when maximally flexed allows assessment of the integrity of the ulnar collateral ligament.
    e. A complete examination makes X-rays unnecessary.

41. **Ulnar nerve palsy**:
    a. Ulnar nerve palsy in cyclists is caused by direct pressure on the nerve from the handle bars.
    b. The site of injury is usually the arcade of Froche.
    c. Foam padding and alterations of hand positions on the handlebars have no effect in preventing cyclist's ulnar nerve palsy.
    d. All the motor and sensory divisions of the ulnar nerve are affected.
    e. Ulnar nerve palsy in cyclists is a relatively recent sports injury, resulting from the newer, lighter-framed bikes.

42. **Keinbock's disease:**
    a. Keinbock's disease is caused by vascular necrosis of the scaphoid bone.
    b. It is an overuse injury.
    c. It can mimic a Guyon's canal syndrome.
    d. Negative radial variance predisposes to Kienbock's disease.
    e. Conservative cast immobilization usually resolves the injury.

43. **Osteitis pubis:**
    a. Osteitis pubis is common in those who participate in jumping sports.
    b. It is often accompanied by a decreased range of hip movements.
    c. It is easily distinguished from a Gilmore's groin.
    d. Negative plain radiology and positive triple-phase bone scanning is pathognomonic of osteitis pubis syndrome.
    e. Spontaneous remission rarely occurs.

44. **Plantar fasciitis:**
    a. The pain associated with plantar fasciitis is usually caused by a local calcanial spur.
    b. Plantar fasciitis is usually associated with progressive heel pain during the day.
    c. It is usually relieved by rest.
    d. It may be treated with a shock-absorbing heel pad.
    e. It is associated with pes cavus.

45. **Osgood–Schlatter's disease:**
    a. Osgood–Schlatter's disease is caused by inflammation of the patellar tendon insertion into the inferior pole of the patella.
    b. It usually occurs during a rapid growth period.
    c. It is usually caused by an acute injury.
    d. It is associated with patella alta.
    e. It rarely requires surgery.

46. **Olecranon impingement syndrome:**
    a. The olecranon impingement syndrome is an overuse syndrome caused by repetitive valvus extension overloading, which results in local trauma to the olecranon process.
    b. Olecranon impingement syndrome is very common in boxers.
    c. Pain often develops while extending the elbow during a throwing motion.
    d. Radiology may show hypertrophy of the olecranon and spurring of the olecranon tip.
    e. Alteration of throwing mechanics is a feature in preventing a recurrence.

47. **Burner syndrome (brachial plexus injury):**
    a. Burner syndrome can occur in up to 50 per cent of American football players.
    b. It usually affects the middle and lower trunks of the brachial plexus.
    c. Electromyography is warranted if burner symptoms do not resolve within 48 hours.
    d. The supraspinatus, deltoid and biceps muscles are frequently weak on clinical examination.
    e. Resistance rehabilitation forms the cornerstone of treatment for neurogenic muscle weakness following a burner syndrome.

48. **Blow-out fractures of the orbit:**
    a. Blow-out fractures usually occur following a direct blow to the eye.
    b. The superior and lateral margins of the orbit are most often damaged.
    c. A blow against a closed glottis often identifies a previously undetected orbital fracture.
    d. Soft tissue bulging and loose bony fragments are almost always visible on X-ray.
    e. The upper maxillary sinus margin is usually distorted.

49. **Malignant brain oedema syndrome:**
    a. Malignant brain oedema syndrome occurs in adult and elderly athletes.
    b. It occurs as a consequence of head trauma.
    c. It sometimes results in death.
    d. It is associated with little brain swelling and a large degree of brain injury.
    e. Fatal neurological outcome is usually secondary to the initial brain injury.

Musculoskeletal medicine

50. **Q angle:**
    a. The Q angle is measured by determining the centre point of the patella and drawing a line to the anterior superior iliac spine proximally, and through the tibial tubercle distally.
    b. Normal Q angles range from 8–10° in females and 12–16° in males.
    c. A decreased Q angle is associated with patellar subluxation.
    d. The Q angle may be reduced by orthotics in standing subjects (research indicates that orthotics have no effect on the Q angle in moving subjects).
    e. When the knee joint is extended, the vastus medialis muscle counteracts the tendency of the patella to displace laterally.

51. **Carpal tunnel syndrome:**
    a. The incidence of carpal tunnel syndrome (CTS) in the general population is 4 per cent, but it rarely occurs in athletes.
    b. A positive Tinnel's sign is pathopneumonic of a carpal tunnel syndrome.
    c. Phalen's sign is usually positive.
    d. Pain may be experienced in the forearm and shoulder.
    e. The first one and a half ulnar digits are rarely involved.

52. **Lateral epicondylitis:**
    a. Over 80 per cent of steroid injections relieve painful symptoms.
    b. Less than 50 per cent of oral NSAIDs are effective in relieving symptoms.
    c. In 80 per cent of cases physiotherapy ultra sound treatments will relieve symptoms.
    d. Elbow straps should not be worn in the acute phase.
    e. Rehabilitation should be started within 48 hours of steroid injection.

53. **Chronic low back pain (CLBP):**
    a. Co-ordination training is less effective than endurance training for sufferers of CLBP.
    b. Back muscle weakness is considered as levels below 64 per cent of the body weight.
    c. Extensor trunk muscles are usually stronger than flexor trunk muscles.
    d. Over 93 per cent of western athletes suffer from low back pain.
    e. Runners are the commonest athletic group to suffer CLBP.

54. **Achilles tendon injuries:**
    a. Three-quarters of Achilles tendon injuries in competitive athletes are paratendonitis.
    b. Females are more prone to Achilles tendon injuries.
    c. Excessive ankle dorsiflexion has an aetiological role in Achilles tendon injuries.
    d. The usual composition of the Achilles tendon is 30 per cent elastin, 21 per cent collagen and 58 per cent water.
    e. Animal studies suggest that the Achilles tendon adapts to exercise by decreasing its total weight.

55. **Legg–Calve–Perthes disease:**
    a. Legg–Calve–Perthes disease presents as a painful limp after activity.
    b. Pain is always localized to the hip.
    c. Legg–Calve–Perthes disease usually presents between the ages of 4 and 8 years.
    d. The incidence is higher in boys than girls.
    e. Magnetic resonance imaging is effective in detecting early, preclinical or asymptomatic avascular necrosis, and can help to localize the extent of the bone necrosis.

56. **The rotator cuff syndrome:**
    a. The rotator cuff syndrome is associated with a positive Spurling's test.
    b. It is associated with limited shoulder abduction.
    c. It is associated with a negative Stoddard's test.
    d. It is associated with a negative Hawkin's test.
    e. It is associated with a positive Near's test.

57. **Patellofemoral syndrome:**
    a. Chondromalacia patellae refers to non-degenerative patellofemoral syndrome.
    b. The patella improves the overall effectiveness of knee flexion.
    c. Two and one half times the body weight is placed on the patellofemoral joint when ascending stairs.
    d. Cyrano-shaped patellae are associated with a reduced incidence of patellofemoral syndrome.
    e. Surface degeneration of the patellar cartilage is commonly seen with advancing years.

58. **Heel spurs:**
    a. Heel spurs are present in up to 30 per cent of the asymptomatic population.
    b. They are present in up to 75 per cent of athletes with plantar fasciitis.
    c. The calcaneal spur is usually a result of traction stresses acting through the plantar fascia onto its origin at the calcaneous.
    d. Exercise-related heel spurs are usually large and fluffy in appearance.
    e. Large heel spurs are usually a cause of pain.

59. **Morton's metatarsalgia:**
    a. This usually occurs in association with a hallux valgus deformity.
    b. Pain is usually at the second or third intermetatarsal space.
    c. Carbamazepine is helpful in reducing the symptom of pain.
    d. The symptoms of Morton's metatarsalgia are made worse by removing the shoes.
    e. Pathological examination of a Morton's nodule reveals that it usually consists of fibrous rather than neural tissue.

60. **Iliopsoas injury:**
    a. An iliopsoas muscle injury is the most common source of groin pain in soccer players.
    b. Iliopsoas injury is usually caused by direct trauma at the musculo-tendinous junction.
    c. Pain is elicited by active hip extension against resistance.
    d. The pain is usually located at the level of the pubic tubercle.
    e. Iliopsoas muscle injury is a cause of the perforating nerve syndrome.

61. **Fractures associated with inversional injuries of the ankle joint:**
    a. Twisting ankle injuries are associated with fractures of the calcanium.
    b. Twisting ankle injuries are associated with longitudinal fractures of the long axis of the fifth metatarsal.
    c. Twisting ankle injuries are associated with fractures of the upper fibula.
    d. Twisting ankle injuries are associated with a Maissoneuve fracture.
    e. Twisting ankle injuries are associated with osteochondral fractures of the dome of the talus.

62. **Salter–Harris fractures:**
    a. Salter–Harris fracture classification relates to fractures involving the growth plate of unfused skeletons, and is based on the clinical importance of the injury.
    b. Salter–Harris type 5 injuries are easily identified on plain radiographs.
    c. Prognosis of a Salter–Harris type 1 fracture is very good.
    d. Salter–Harris type 1 injuries are easily identified on plain radiographs.
    e. A Salter–Harris type 2 fracture involves injury through the metaphysis and into the epiphyseal plate.

63. **Avulsion fractures:**
    a. Avulsion of the anterior inferior iliac spine is due to excessive muscle contraction by the sartorius muscle.
    b. Anterior superior iliac spine avulsion is usually caused by excessive contraction of the rectus femorus muscle.
    c. In younger individuals, avulsion of the medial epicondyle may be misinterpreted as a normal trochlear ossification centre.
    d. An avulsion fracture of the ischial tuberosity is caused by the chronic stress of the pull of the adductor longus muscle.
    e. An avulsion fracture is an injury resulting in a displacement of a bony fragment from the parent bone; it always occurs at the site of a tendinous insertion.

64. **Bennett's fracture:**
    a. A Bennett's fracture occurs at the base of the thumb, and often involves damage to the joint surface.
    b. Swelling and discoloration usually occur at the DIP joint.
    c. A Bennett's fracture can be caused by overuse, and is regularly seen in rowers.
    d. It is easily differentiated from a scaphoid fracture.
    e. It is caused by a fall onto the outstretched hand.

65. **Ulnar collateral ligament injuries of the elbow:**
    a. Ulnar collateral ligament injuries are caused by repetitive varus stresses increasing tension on the ulnar lateral collateral ligament.
    b. Injury to the flexor and pronator muscles of the elbow and forearm increases the stresses on the ulnar collateral ligament
    c. Ulnar collateral ligament injuries can be associated with an ulnar neuropathy at the elbow.
    d. Surgical reconstruction of the ulnar collateral ligament usually involves autografting of the palmaris longus or plantares tendons.
    e. Throwing and racket sports are the most common offenders in causing ulnar collateral ligament. injuries.

66. **Spondylolysis:**
    a. Spondylolysis is best observed on a lateral radiograph.
    b. Spondylolysis affects approximately 1 per cent of the North American population.
    c. It is caused by a stress fracture to the transverse process.
    d. The L4 level is the most commonly affected site.
    e. Less than half of patients with spondylolysis will develop spondylolisthesis.

67. **Acromioclavicular injuries:**
    a. The acromioclavicular joint is the site of the most commonly encountered shoulder dislocation.
    b. Type 6 injuries occur when the patient's clavicle is displaced inferiorly to the coracoid process.
    c. Type 3 acromioclavicular separation injuries show complete tearing of the acromioclavicular and coracoclavicular ligaments, with resulting dislocation of the acromioclavicular joint.
    d. Type 1 sprains involve a partial disruption of the acromioclavicular ligament and capsule.
    e. Alexander views of the shoulder are required to diagnose type 4 dislocations.

68. **Patellofemoral pain:**
    a. Non-operative treatment of patellofemoral pain succeeds in up to 80 per cent of cases.
    b. Surgical options should only be considered after 6 months of failed conservative treatment.
    c. Patellofemoral syndrome refers to a specific pathology.
    d. Patellofemoral syndrome usually presents with an acute, persisting, sharp pain, exacerbated by going up and down stairs.
    e. Patients with a previous history of Osgood–Schlatter's disease have an increased risk of later developing patellofemoral syndrome.

69. **Malalignments associated with the patellofemoral syndrome: These include the following:**
    a. Increased Q angle.
    b. Spondylolisthesis.
    c. Tight lateral retinaculum.
    d. Pes cavus.
    e. Atrophy of the vastus medialis oblique muscle.

70. **Levator scapula syndrome:**
    a. The levator scapula originates on the transverse process of the cervical vertebrae C1–C7, and has a broad insertion onto the supero-medial border of the scapula.
    b. The patient usually complains of specific periscapular pain.
    c. Levator scapula syndrome is frequently exacerbated by sailing and golfing.
    d. The levator scapula syndrome is amenable to local steroid injection with the patient in a prone position supporting the weight of his or her body on abducted elbows approximately shoulder-width apart.
    e. Levator scapula syndrome must be differentiated from gall bladder disease and pancreatitis.

71. **Popliteal tendonitis:**
    a. The popliteus works synergistically with the anterior cruciate ligament to prevent anterior displacement at the femur.
    b. Popliteal tendon injuries are more common following downhill running.
    c. The ligaments of Winslow form part of the lateral origin of the popliteus muscle.
    d. The patient may present with posterior knee pain on descending stairs.
    e. Palpation of the popliteal tendon is best achieved by placing the patient's leg on the examiner's shoulder.

Special groups

72. **The young athlete:**
    a. Ligaments in young athletes are weaker than neighbouring cartilage and bone.
    b. Following a significant supination inversion injury to the ankle joint, the young athlete is more likely to sustain a bone or epiphyseal fracture of the lateral malleolus than an anterior talo-fibular ligament tear.
    c. In the young athlete, a significant injury to the anterior cruciate ligament may result in an avulsion of the ligament and bone complex rather than rupture of the ligament.
    d. Iselin's disease is a traction apophysitis at the base of the 5th metatarsal that can occur in skeletally immature athletes.
    e. Sever's disease is typically seen at the age of 14 years in boys and 13 years in girls.

73. **Exercise and ageing:**
    a. As we age, peak performance endurance activity decreases by 1–2 per cent per year, starting in the late twenties.
    b. VO_2 max decreases by about 2 per cent per decade, starting in the third decade for women and the fourth decade for men.
    c. The respiratory vital capacity and forced expiratory volume decrease linearly with age.
    d. The total lung capacity increases with age.
    e. The residual volume increases with age.

74. **Osteochondritis dissecans:**
    a. Osteochondritis dissecans of the knee is a disorder in which a fragment of cartilage and subchondral bone separates from an articular surface.
    b. Osteochondritis dissecans is usually caused by trauma.
    c. The Wilson test confirms the diagnosis of osteochrondritis dissecans of the lateral femoral condyle.
    d. Antero-posterior and lateral radiographs confirm the diagnosis in most cases.
    e. The prognosis of osteochrondritis dissecans is better in older, rather than younger, athletes.

75. **Exercise in diabetes: Proven benefits include the following:**
    a. Increased insulin sensitivity.
    b. Reduced coronary risk.
    c. Improved self-esteem and self-confidence.
    d. Improved lipid profile.
    e. Decreased haemoglobin A1.

76. **Absolute contraindications for exercise during pregnancy: These include the following:**
    a. Ruptured membranes.
    b. Placenta praevia.
    c. Palpitations or irregular heart rhythms.
    d. High blood pressure.
    e. Anaemia.

77. **Female incontinence and exercise:**
    a. Women are as likely as men to be incontinent during exercise.
    b. Upwards of 40 per cent of all women report some degree of incontinence during exercise.
    c. High impact exercise results in more episodes of incontinence than low impact exercise.
    d. The number of vaginal deliveries does not correlate positively with incontinence during exercise.
    e. Over 40 per cent of female weight-lifters experience incontinence during activity.

78. **Restrictive eating behaviour: Common physical symptoms and signs include the following:**
    a. Diarrhoea.
    b. Tachycardia.
    c. Hypothermia.
    d. Brittle hair and nails.
    e. Heat intolerance.

79. **Restrictive eating behaviour: Common laboratory findings include the following:**
    a. Elevated follicle stimulating hormone (FSH) levels.
    b. Normal luteinizing hormone (LH) levels.
    c. Normal T3, T4 and TSH values.
    d. Hyponatraemia.
    e. Proteinuria.

80. **Pregnancy and exercise:**
    a. There is a definite association between elevated maternal temperature during pregnancy and the incidence of congenital malformations in the foetus.
    b. Splanchnic blood flow decreases to a level of 40 per cent of resting levels during athletic training.
    c. High intensity exercise may impair the nutrients and oxygen available to the embryo or foetus due to a reduction in splanchnic circulation.
    d. There is an increased incidence of musculoskeletal injury during pregnancy.
    e. The intensity of exercise during pregnancy should be limited to a heart rate of less than 140 beats/minute for a duration of less than 15 minutes.

81. **Rugby union injuries:**
    a. The neck is the most commonly injured site.
    b. The back row and scrum halves are the most commonly injured players.
    c. Rugby union players are likely to be injured one in every three times they participate in their sport.
    d. Professional rugby is likely to have a lower injury incidence than recreational or amateur rugby football.
    e. Acromioclavicular joint injuries are the most common shoulder injury among rugby players.

82. **Skateboarding:**
   a. The most common skateboarding injury is lateral ankle ligament tears.
   b. The radius and ulna are the most commonly fractured bones.
   c. The majority of skateboard deaths involve accidents with motor vehicles.
   d. Three per cent of skateboarding injuries involve motor vehicles.
   e. 'Goofy foot' is a skateboard specific overuse injury of the 5th metatarsal.

83. **Head injuries in soccer:**
   a. Head injuries account for 25 per cent of all soccer-related injuries.
   b. Younger players are more susceptible to skull injuries.
   c. The symptoms of soccer-related head injuries can include insomnia and impaired memory.
   d. The mechanisms of head injuries in soccer include head-to-head contact.
   e. Professional soccer players head the ball on average five times in a game.
   f. Goalkeepers never experience head injuries, as they do not head the ball.

84. **Breaststroker's knee:**
   a. Breaststroker's knee commonly involves the pes anserina bursa.
   b. It regularly involves the tibial attachment of the medial collateral ligament of the knee.
   c. It never affects the medial meniscus.
   d. It is an activity-specific injury.
   e. It is caused by an acute macro-trauma.

85. **Snowboarding injuries**
   a. Snowboarders have a similar injury rate to Alpine skiers.
   b. Upper limb injuries are more common than lower limb injuries among snowboarders.
   c. The wearing of hard shell boots gives greater protection to the knees of snowboarders.
   d. A direct blow is the most commonly encountered mechanism of injury.
   e. The most common snowboard accident is a collision.

86. **Physiological function and ageing:**
   a. Maximum oxygen uptake declines at a rate of 1 per cent per year after the third decade of life.
   b. Isometric and dynamic muscle strength begins to decrease after the fifth decade of life.
   c. The ageing process is the cause for the decline in the aerobic and anaerobic exercise capacities noted with advancing years.
   d. The geriatric (over 65 years) population will account for more than 20 per cent of the total population of North America in the year 2030.
   e. There is a slow decline in loss of lean tissue after the age of 65.

87. **Frostbite:**
   a. Frostbite usually occurs at a skin temperature of 11 to 12°C.
   b. Preventative measures include wearing tight stockings.
   c. Frostbite is more common in cigarette smokers.
   d. Frostbite is caused by freezing of extracellular water and dehydration damage to the exposed skin.
   e. The immediate treatment for frostbite is re-warming of the affected area, and this should be maintained over the following 48 hours.

88. **Resistance training for the middle-aged adult:**
   a. Thirty per cent of a projected maximum lift is an appropriate starting weight for a resistance activity.
   b. Eighty per cent of a predicted maximum lift is an appropriate starting weight for a resistance activity.
   c. Isometric exercises are appropriate for patients with left ventricular decompensation.
   d. Dynamic large muscle, low resistance, high repetition exercises are the most appropriate for the middle-aged individual.
   e. Incremental increases in the resistance should be of the order of 3–5 per cent in the progressive phase of a resistance rehabilitation exercise.

Exercise prescription

89. **Endurance exercise:**
    a. Endurance training results in an increase in the age-related decline in circulation T cell function and related cytokine production.
    b. Endurance exercise can be associated with an increase in LDL-cholesterol.
    c. Endurance exercise can be associated with an increase in HDL2-cholesterol.
    d. Prolonged endurance exercise causes a reduction in circulating aldosterone.
    e. Prolonged endurance exercise can cause a physiological anaemia.

90. **Proper bicycle fit:**
    a. Proper frame size allows a 2.5–5 cm between the cyclist's crotch and the top frame tube in the standing position.
    b. The correct seat height for a cyclist is determined by a tibial-femoral angle in the seated position of 20–30°.
    c. The correct handlebar to saddle reach is the distance between the elbow joint and the extended fingers.
    d. Seat position is determined by placing the pedals at the 3 o'clock and 9 o'clock positions. A line drawn from the from the forward knee should dissect the middle of the pedal.
    e. The handlebar height should be at a level of 7.5 cm above the saddle height.

91. **Normal hormonal responses to exercise:**
    a. Growth hormone release is increased during prolonged exercise.
    b. Insulin and glucagon secretion is increased during prolonged exercise.
    c. Norepinephrine and epinephrine are both increased during prolonged exercise.
    d. Cortisol and growth hormone variations during exercise are in proportion to the intensity of exercise.
    e. Growth hormone response to exercise returns to baseline once the exercise stimulus has been withdrawn.

92. **Exercise for weight loss:**
    a. Jogging for 15 minutes daily, 3 days a week is the most efficient method for weight loss in obese subjects.
    b. Walking 20–30 minutes daily, 5–7 days weekly at a low to moderate intensity is the most efficient method for weight loss in obese subjects.
    c. High repetition resistance exercise 3 days a week is the most efficient method for weight loss in obese subjects.
    d. Lack of motivation is a significant factor in the drop-out rate for obese individuals on an exercise programme.
    e. Intensity of exercise is the single most important element in a weight loss exercise programme.

93. **Resistance exercise:**
    a. An isokinetic activity is one that occurs at a constant angular velocity with a variable resistance.
    b. Isokinetic resistance exercise programmes have been shown to be superior to isometric and isotonic with respect to endurance and strength improvement.
    c. Motivation is generally superior with isotonic exercise.
    d. Muscle endurance and strength is developed more effectively through isotonic rather than isometric exercise.
    e. Isometric training produces a more uniform development of strength.

Drugs, supplements and toxicology

94. **Alcohol:**
    a. Alcohol is exclusively metabolized by the enzyme alcohol dehydrogenase in the liver.
    b. Acute alcohol ingestion does not affect physiological function.
    c. The 'hangover' effect of alcohol significantly reduces anaerobic performance.
    d. Alcohol metabolism shifts the lactate peruvate ratio.
    e. Beer is a reasonable source of carbohydrate.

95. **Erythropoietin:**
    a. Erythropoietin (EPO) abuse is suggested by a haematocrit count greater than 0.52.
    b. DNA recombinant human erythropoietin (rEPO) can increase haemoglobin concentration, but has no effect on maximum oxygen uptake.
    c. rEPO is classified as a doping substance by the International Skiing Federation, but is allowed by the International Olympic Committee.
    d. rEPO cannot be detected in the urine and serum of humans.
    e. rEPO can be screened indirectly by determining trans receptors in blood.

96. **Prohibited substances: The following drugs are prohibited by the International Olympic Committee:**
    a. Domperidone.
    b. Morphine.
    c. Terbutaline.
    d. Fenoterol.
    e. Phenylpropanolamine.

97. **Steroid injections:**
    a. Corticosteroids produce an anti-inflammatory effect by altering thymocyte activity.
    b. Repeated joint injections increase the possibility of cortisone arthropathies.
    c. Soluble preparations such as betamethasone must never be injected into the carpal tunnel.
    d. Trimcinolone injection of a tennis elbow is rarely associated with post-injection pain.
    e. The injured area should be exercised in the first 24 hours post-injection.

98. **Alcohol:**
    a. Alcohol is a contributory factor in at least 60 per cent of all boating fatalities.
    b. Acute alcohol ingestion improves hand–eye co-ordination.
    c. Alcohol may precipitate cardiac arrhythmia in the susceptible individual.
    d. Athletes in general drink more coffee than alcohol.
    e. Alcohol is considered an ergogenic drug.

99. **Restricted drugs in sport:**
    a. Iron supplements are prohibited by the International Olympic Committee (IOC).
    b. Caffeine is prohibited for selected Olympic sports.
    c. Alcohol is allowed for all Olympic sports.
    d. Salbutamol is a substance prohibited by the IOC.
    e. Piroxicam is prohibited for selected Olympic sports.

100. **Mineral/iron supplementation:**
    a. Supplementing with oral iron in the non-anaemic state will improve physiological performance.
    b. The recommended daily intake for iron is 10 mg for men and 50 mg for women.
    c. Iron derived from plant food (non-haem iron) is better absorbed than iron derived from animal foods.
    d. Iron supplementation should be recommended for all exercising athletes.
    e. The most common side effects of iron supplementation are nausea and constipation.

101. **Growth hormone:**
    a. Human growth hormone (HGH) supplements in non-deficient adults can increase lean body mass.
    b. Human growth hormone supplements increase skeletal muscle mass and strength.
    c. Human growth hormone abuse is associated with Creutzfeldt–Jakob disease.
    d. Human growth hormone abuse is a relatively recent phenomenon.
    e. Growth hormone (GH) is a banned substance, but growth hormone releasing factor (GHRF) is not banned by the IOC or the NCAA.

102. **Protein:**
    a. The recommended daily intake for a competitive 90 kg (~ 200 lb) athlete is 160 gm of protein per day.
    b. Protein is rarely used as an energy source during endurance exercise.
    c. All vegetarian athletes require protein supplements.
    d. Forty per cent of an athlete's diet should be made up of protein.
    e. Low fat, high carbohydrate diets with a low protein content often leave the athlete deficient in folic acid.

103. **Ergolytic drugs: The following are classified as ergolytic drugs:**
    a. Alcohol.
    b. Marijuana.
    c. Salbutamol.
    d. Diuretics.
    e. Propranolol.

104. **Chromium:**
    a. Hexavalent chromium is highly toxic and may be carcinogenic.
    b. The recommended daily allowance (RDA) of chromium is 50–200 mg.
    c. Chromium picolinate can increase lean body mass and reduce body fat percentage in association with resistance
    d. The body's chromium requirements increase with exercise.

105. **Zinc:**
   a. The recommended daily intake of zinc for males is 15 mg.
   b. Normal serum zinc levels are between 5 and 15 mg/dl.
   c. The average 2850 calorie American diet easily meets the recommended daily intake of zinc.
   d. Zinc deficiencies are common in a distance running athlete.
   e. Green vegetables are the best source of dietary zinc.

106. **Antioxidants:**
   a. Oral, Superoxide Dismutase (SOD), supplementation reduces muscle cell injury following exercise.
   b. Oral cysteine supplementation can increase body glutathione production.
   c. The recommended daily allowance of vitamin E is 10 mg.
   d. Oral vitamin A is associated with significant side effects.
   e. Vitamin C assists in regeneration of vitamin E following its antioxidant action.

107. **Carbohydrates:**
   a. Carbohydrates are stored in limited quantities in the liver and muscles as glycogen.
   b. Reduced carbohydrate stores result in protein gluco-neogenesis during prolonged endurance exercise.
   c. Reduced carbohydrate metabolism results in ketosis.
   d. The brain uses blood glucose exclusively as a fuel.
   e. Sixty per cent of the daily calorie intake of an exercising individual should be in the form of simple carbohydrates.

108. **Melatonin:**
   a. Melatonin is secreted by the pineal gland.
   b. Melatonin can help with mild sleep disorders.
   c. Scientific evidence confirms its ability to fight jet lag.
   d. Side effects include early morning awakening and vivid dreams.
   e. 40 mg of melatonin 1 hour before bed time is the recommended dose for moderate sleep disorders.

109. **The phosphagens:**
    a. ATP and phosphocreatine are collectively referred to as the phosphagens.
    b. The total muscular stores of phosphagens in females is very small.
    c. Sprinting flat out through 200 m would probably empty the phosphagen stores.
    d. Kicking a football utilizes stored phosphagens as the primary energy source.
    e. There are higher stored levels of phosphagen in male subjects.

Anatomy

110. **Axillary nerve:**
    a. Axillary nerve injury results in weakness in shoulder adduction.
    b. Axillary nerve injury can occur secondary to shoulder dislocation.
    c. Electromyographic changes of denervation are usually observed in the deltoid muscle 4 weeks post-injury.
    d. Axillary nerve palsy causes injury of the scapula.
    e. Sensory changes are often noted in the upper outer shoulder following injury.

111. **Fracture at the base of the 5th metatarsal:**
    a. Fracture at the base of the 5th metatarsal may result from an eversional injury of the ankle.
    b. Fracture at the base of the 5th metatarsal results from avulsion of the insertion of the peroneus brevis tendon.
    c. Fracture at the base of the 5th metatarsal usually results in a fracture line transverse to the long axis of the metatarsal.
    d. An unfused apophysis usually lies longitudinal to the long axis of the metatarsal, and can therefore easily be distinguished from a fracture at the base of the 5th metatarsal.

112. **Scaphoid fractures:**
    a. The easiest time to see a scaphoid fracture on a plain X-ray is within the first 12 hours post-injury.
    b. The proximal pole of the scaphoid is the commonest site of fracture and it carries the highest risk of avascular necrosis.
    c. The distal pole of the scaphoid is fractured in 10 per cent of cases and runs no risk of avascular necrosis.
    d. Bone resorption around a fractured scaphoid improves the chances of visualizing a scaphoid fracture.
    e. Ninety per cent of carpal bone fractures are through the scaphoid.

113. **Acromioclavicular joint subluxation:**
   a. Acromioclavicular joint subluxation is the most common rugby-related shoulder injury.
   b. The width of the normal acromioclavicular joint is usually less than 10 mm in adults.
   c. In normal individuals, the inferior surface of the acromium and the clavicle should be in a straight line on antero-posterior X-rays.
   d. Separation of greater than 1 cm in adults signifies a subluxation of the acromioclavicular joint.
   e. Bilateral weight-bearing views are essential to identify an acromioclavicular subluxation.

114. **The vastus medialis muscle:**
   a. The vastus medialis muscle is enervated by the tibial nerve.
   b. Its root enervation is L5, S1, S2.
   c. The muscle can be activated by flexing the knee.
   d. Vastus medialis oblique atrophy can occur as a consequence of an L3, 4 disc prolapse.
   e. Vastus medialis atrophy is commonly associated with subluxing patella syndrome.

115. **The supraspinatus muscle:**
   a. The supraspinatus muscle is enervated by the dorsal scapular nerve.
   b. It is commonly affected in middle trunk brachial plexus injuries.
   c. The supraspinatus tendon is inserted into the greater tuberosity of the humerus.
   d. The supraspinatus muscle is an external rotator of the arm.
   e. It receives the majority of its enervation from the C7 nerve root level.

116. **The adductor longus:**
   a. The adductor longus takes its origin from the inferior ramus of the pubis.
   b. It is enervated by the femoral nerve.
   c. It adducts the hip.
   d. It is commonly injured by rugby half-backs and hockey players.
   e. It may be compromised by an obturator nerve lesion.

Cardiology and sport

117. **Lone atrial fibrillation:**
    a. Lone atrial fibrillation always occurs with hyperthyroidism.
    b. Lone atrial fibrillation can always be prevented by avoiding triggering factors.
    c. Class 1A anti-arrhythmogenic agents are unhelpful in treating lone nature fibrillation.
    d. Lone atrial fibrillation patients run the risk of subsequent stroke.
    e. Atrial fibrillation is a contraindication for vigorous athletic activity.

118. **Common rhythm disturbances: Common rhythm disturbances seen in resting ECGs of athletes include the following:**
    a. Sinus bradycardia.
    b. Mobitz type 2.
    c. Mobitz type 1.
    d. First degree heart block.
    e. Junctional rhythms.

119. **The athletic heart syndrome: ECG changes commonly observed in the athletic heart syndrome include the following:**
    a. Decreased P wave amplitude.
    b. Left ventricular hypertrophy.
    c. Tall peaked T waves in the limb and precordial leads.
    d. T wave inversion in the precordial leads only.
    e. SE segment elevation.

120. **Marfan's syndrome: This may be suspected in a 190 cm (~6 ft 4 in) 16-year-old boy under the following circumstances:**
    a. If there is a mid-systolic click audible on oscillation of the precordium.
    b. If he is myopic.
    c. If he shows antero-thoracic deformity.
    d. If his upper to lower body ratio is more than one standard deviation below the mean.
    e. If his arm span is greater than his height.

121. **Hypertrophic cardiomyopathy in the athletic population:**
   a. This is the most common cause of sudden death in a sports setting in subjects under the age of 40 years.
   b. It is associated with a jerky, sustained pulse.
   c. It is associated with a third heart sound.
   d. It is occasionally associated with a late systolic murmur.
   e. It may be associated with a double apical impulse on palpation of the precordium.

122. **Aortic insufficiency and exercise:**
   a. Cardiac murmurs can be detected in up to 85 per cent of athletes who participate in dynamic sports.
   b. Aortic insufficiency is associated with a systolic ejection murmur in the aortic area.
   c. Aortic insufficiency is associated with prolonged asymptomatic phases.
   d. Symptomatic athletes with mild aortic regurgitation and no left ventricular hypertrophy are safe to participate in competitive sport.
   e. Asymptomatic athletes with severe aortic regurgitation and a normal left ventricle can safely participate in sport.

Exercise physiology

123. **Functional aerobic impairment:**
   a. Functional aerobic impairment (FAI) is the percentage by which an individual's functional capacity falls below that expected for his/her age, sex and conditioning state.
   b. The percentage FAI is equal to a predicted VO_2 max value minus the observed VO_2 max value divided by the predicted VO_2 max value.
   c. An FAI of greater than 68 per cent implies extreme impairment.
   d. Haemoglobinopathy can increase percentage FAI.
   e. Beta-adrenergic blockade has no effect on percentage FAI.

124. **Second wind:**
   a. A 'second wind' is due to improved contractility of the diaphragm.
   b. It is due to changes in diaphragmatic blood flow.
   c. It is due to increased circulating catecholamines.
   d. There is increased recruitment of the accessory muscles of respiration.
   e. There are no lung volume changes associated with second wind.

125. **Muscle contractions:**
   a. An isotonic muscle contraction results in muscle shortening while developing tension.
   b. An isokinetic muscle contraction results in the muscle developing tension but not changing in length.
   c. An isometric muscle contraction results in the muscle shortening while developing maximal tension throughout the full range of movement at a constant speed.
   d. An eccentric muscle contraction results in muscle lengthening while developing tension.
   e. A concentric muscle contraction results in muscle shortening while developing tension.

126. **Fast twitch motor units:**
    a. Fast twitch motor units have a high anaerobic capacity and a low aerobic capacity.
    b. They have a high capillary density.
    c. They have a slow contraction time.
    d. They have a rapid fatigue ability.
    e. They have a high force of contraction.

127. **Sleep and exercise:**
    a. The over-training syndrome primarily occurs because of insufficient rest.
    b. Over-trained athletes become progressively more susceptible to infection.
    c. Insomnia is one of the cardinal signs of the over-training syndrome.
    d. Six and a half hours' sleep is adequate for the exercising athlete.
    e. The over-training syndrome can be cured by increasing daily sleeping to 9½ h nightly.

128. **Aerobic and anaerobic energy system contributions during sporting activities:**
    a. 800 m running has a similar contribution from the aerobic and anaerobic energy systems.
    b. Swinging a golf club has little or no call on the aerobic system of energy production.
    c. Basketball derives 90 per cent of its energy from the aerobic energy production system.
    d. Rowing 200 m is a predominantly aerobic activity.
    e. Skating 10 000 m derives only 10 per cent of energy from the anaerobic system.

129. **Sleep:**
    a. Daily sleep duration is directly associated with all causes of mortality.
    b. Individuals who sleep more than 10 hours per day have an elevated mortality risk.
    c. Individuals who sleep less than 5 hours per night have a reduced mortality risk.
    d. Individuals who sleep 7 hours per night have a reduced mortality rate.
    e. Resting sympathetic nerve activity is increased after a bout of endurance training.

130. **Physiological assessment:**
    a. The Kline test is a functional assessment of anaerobic capacity.
    b. The Lusbera shuttle run test is functional assessment of aerobic capacity.
    c. Cooper's 12-minute test correlates aerobic capicity with the distance travelled in a 20-minute run/walk test.
    d. The Ergo Jump test assesses the power output of the quadriceps musculature.
    e. There is a direct correlation between the Sergeant jump test and the 40 m dash.

131. **Ozone and exercise:**
    a. Reduction in exercise performance has been observed when exercising at the relatively low ozone pollutant level of 0.18 ppm.
    b. Prolonged exposure to ozone levels of 0.08 ppm can induce changes in lung function.
    c. Ozone exposure has a most significant effect on pulmonary and cardiovascular performance in cardiac patients.
    d. Indomethacin partially blocks ozone-induced respiratory symptoms.
    e. Ozone exposure often can mimic the symptoms of acute myocardial infarction.

132. **Metabolic equivalents (METs):**
    a. A metabolic equivalent unit is approximately equal to 3.5 ml of oxygen consumed per kg of body weight per minute.
    b. METs equal the resting metabolic rate.
    c. The metabolic equivalent units are useful in identifying an activity with an appropriate exercise intensity for cardiac rehabilitation patients.
    d. A metabolic equivalent unit can easily be interchanged with a heart rate monitoring approach to exercise intensity monitoring.
    e. Rating of perceived exertion and metabolic equivalent units cannot be directly substituted.

133. **Body composition:**
   a. Body mass index is calculated by dividing the height in metres squared by the body weight in kilograms.
   b. A body mass index of greater than 30 kg/m^2 in a 30-year-old indicates that the individual is obese.
   c. A diagnosis of obesity is confirmed in a 20-year-old athlete if the body fat is greater than 15 per cent.
   d. The average body fat of elite gymnasts is usually less than 8 per cent.
   e. The average body fat of international rugby players is usually in the order of 16 per cent.

Therapy and radiology

134. **Steroid arthropathy:**
    a. Steroid injections are chondro-protective.
    b. Steroid arthropathy usually develops following oral steroid use, in the absence of associated underlying disease.
    c. The ankle and knee joint are the joints most commonly affected by steroid arthropathy.
    d. Alcohol abuse decreases the likelihood of a steroid arthropathy.
    e. Concurrent therapy with non-steroidal anti-inflammatories increases the likelihood of a steroid arthropathy.

135. **Therapeutic cold laser treatment:**
    a. Cold laser treatment reduces the vascularity of wounds.
    b. It affects RNA production.
    c. It reduces mitochondrial activity.
    d. Cold lasers are always visible.
    e. They have no pain relieving effect.

136. **Injection therapy: Relative contraindications for injection therapy include the following:**
    a. Localized cellulitis.
    b. An unco-operative patient.
    c. An acute injury.
    d. Previous site injections of greater than 160 mg of steroid.
    e. Diabetes.

137. **Shoulder radiology:**
    a. Antero-posterior (AP) views can easily demonstrate Hill–Sachs lesions and bony Bankart lesions.
    b. AP views can visualize osteoarthritis at the gleno-humeral joint.
    c. Three-view procedures adequately screen for both soft tissue and bony pathology around the shoulder.
    d. A supraspinatus outlet view aids in the diagnosis of rotator cuff injuries by demonstrating the shape of the acromion.
    e. Rotator cuff tears are most common in patients who have a flattened appearance of their acromion.

Part II Answers

General medicine

1. Cluster headaches:

a. False b. False c. True d. False e. False

Cluster headaches are vascular type headaches, which have a temporal distribution. There is male predominance, in comparison to migraine headaches, which have female predominance. The headache is usually unilateral, and commonly affects the eye or the area around it. The patient describes the pain of a cluster headache as boring, stabbing or knife-like. The headache lasts for a short duration (30 minutes–2 hours). There is no prodromal phase, and the nausea and vomiting that frequently accompany migraine headaches are rare. The headaches are severe but benign, and therefore do not preclude participation in contact sports.

Further reading: Bracker, M. D. and Rothrock, J. F. (1989). Cluster headaches among athletes. *Phys. Sports Med.*, **17**, 147.

2. Herpes simplex skin infections:

a. False b. True c. False d. True e. False

Herpes simplex skin infections occur frequently in the sporting fraternity. In rugby football this skin infection is common amongst the forwards, where it is referred to as 'scrum pox'. It is also occurs quite frequently in wrestlers, where it is referred to as herpes gladiatorum. Infections may be recurring, and are usually due to contact with abrasive surfaces, trauma, or sun exposure. The most frequent locations are on the face and hands. The initial attack may be accompanied by pain, adenopathy and fever. The recurrent lesions may be preceded by pruritus or dysaesthesiae.

Prevention of herpes simplex infections amongst contact sports participants can be achieved by very careful attention to hygiene, such as scrubbing of wrestling equipment and headgear. Withdrawing an infected athlete from competitive play is also important, to prevent further spread. Topical acyclovir is often used; however, there is controversy over whether this treatment actually alters the process of the infection once it has passed the vesicular phase. Oral forms of acyclovir may also be used for athletes with recurrent herpes, particularly if the infection causes a large degree of distress or causes a protracted time away from sporting activity. There have been reports in cases of herpes simplex outbreaks where spread to partners has resulted in systemic conditions such as salpingitis.

3. Sudden death in athletes:

a. True b. False c. True d. False e. True

All sport carries a small but definite risk of sudden death, defined as death within 24 hours of the onset of symptoms. Cardiological causes predominate, and these vary with respect to age. Atherosclerotic coronary artery disease is the usual cause of sudden death in individuals over 40 years of age, whereas congenital causes are most common in younger individuals. There is a high incidence of hypertrophic cardiomyopathy, the cause of which is multifactorial. Congenital variations of the ventricular septum, abnormalities of the sympathetic nervous system and inappropriate stimulation of the myocardium have all been implicated. Other causes include valvular heart disease, and non-cardiac causes such as subarachnoid or gastrointestinal haemorrhage.

Further reading: Maron, B. J., Roberts, W. C. and McAllister, H. A. (1980). Sudden death in young athletes. *Circulation*, **62**, 218.

4. Exercise-induced asthma:

a. False b. True c. False d. True e. False

Exercise-induced asthma affects upwards of 15 per cent of the population. It is most commonly reported in individuals who take sporadic exercise. A number of triggering factors are associated with the onset of exercise-induced asthma, including air pollution, cold air, grass, pollen, and a dust-filled environment. The exercise-induced asthma commonly occurs 6–8 minutes into an exercise programme, and may present with wheezing, tightness of the chest, shortness of breath and coughing.

Exercise-induced asthma is caused by inflammation of the bronchial mucosa and submucosa, which causes narrowing of the bronchial airway. The inflammation also causes narrowing of the bronchial airway and hyporeactivity of the bronchial smooth muscles. A diagnosis of exercise-induced asthma is suggested if the peak flow drops by 15 per cent or more after exercise. Exercise-induced asthma can result in a fall in ventilation rate (FVR), which results in a fall in maximum oxygen consumption. Exercised-induced asthma is improved by exercising in a humid environment, such as a swimming pool, and individuals often feel asymptomatic in this setting.

Further reading: Barnes, P. J. (1989). A new approach to the treatment of asthma. *N. Engl. J. Med.*, **321**, 1517–27.

5. Athletic anaemia:

a. False b. True c. False d. True e. False

Endurance-trained athletes tend to have a lower haematocrit and haemoglobin concentration than non-active people, and this apparent abnormality has been called 'athletic anaemia'. This is an inappropriate term, as the alteration in the blood pattern is a normal physiological response to endurance exercise rather than a pathological condition requiring treatment. Regular aerobic exercise expands the plasma volume, which results in dilution of the red blood cells. During vigorous exercise there is an acute loss of plasma volume. This is caused by sweating, increased blood pressure and capillary hydrostatic pressure, and increased osmotic pressure from the increased lactic acid and metabolites of exercising muscle. The body compensates for this by secreting the hormone renin from the kidney; this results in a further release of angiotensen 1 and angiotensen 2, with the subsequent release of aldosterone, which acts on the kidney tubule to resorb sodium and water. Regular exercise therefore results in the expansion of the baseline plasma volume and a dilution of red blood cells. This is a physiological dilution in response to exercise, or a pseudoanaemia.

True anaemias are pathologies requiring specific diagnostic criteria and treatment. Iron-deficiency anaemia is the most common anaemia both in the general population and amongst athletes. Athletes are probably no more prone to iron-deficiency anaemia than non-athletes, although certain sports make them more susceptible. Reduced iron intake has been suggested as a potential risk factor in gymnasts, ballet dancers, distance runners and wrestlers, where a low body weight is advantageous and calorie intake is often reduced. Blood loss is also a potential hazard of athletic activity that may lead to iron-deficiency anaemia. Foot strike haemolysis, caecal slap syndrome and bladder slap syndrome are all reported causes of blood loss in distance runners. Gastrointestinal blood loss is probably the most common cause of iron loss, although this is seldom sufficient to cause iron-deficiency anaemia. In the author's experience, gastrointestinal bleeding secondary to non-steroidal anti-inflammatory use and continued endurance training is the most common cause of iron-deficiency anaemia in athletes.

A diagnosis of iron-deficiency anaemia requires a reduction in haemoglobin and haematocrit to below the reference range, a low MCV, and the presence of hypochromic, microcytic red cells on the blood film. Serum ferritin stores may be low, and the TIBC may be abnormal. Subnormal haemoglobin and haematocrit levels alone are not adequate for a diagnosis of iron-deficiency anaemia.

Many athletes self-dose with iron supplements in a vain attempt to gain a legal edge over fellow competitors. This activity came into prominence following animal research, which showed that iron supplementation in non-anaemic rats improved treadmill times. The research has not been replicated in humans; nevertheless, the practice of oral self-dosing continues and, over the past decades, the incidence of intramuscular and parenteral dosing has increased.

Iron supplementation should be reserved for those individuals with a proven iron-deficiency anaemia. Self-dosing with iron supplements should be actively discouraged, as inappropriate use can lead to significant side effects that will adversely affect both athletic performance and general health. The practice of parenteral iron supplementation should be outlawed; this courts a potential anaphylactic reaction, which can be fatal.

Further reading: Eichner, E. R. (1986). The anemias of athletes. *Phys. Sports Med.*, **14**(9), 122–30.

6. Temperature and exercise:

a. True b. False c. True d. False e. True

Muscle contraction during exercise generates a 20-fold increase in the metabolic rate, and elite athletes may produce over 1000 kcal of heat per hour during activity. During exercise heat production exceeds heat loss, thus producing a rise in the core temperature, which results in an increased skin blood flow and sweating via a hypothalamic response. The core temperature depends on the activity; climatic conditions will affect heat loss. When the external temperature is above 19.8°C, sweating with evaporative cooling is the major mechanism of heat loss; below this temperature, heat loss is by convection and radiation from the skin. These adaptive changes will cause the skin temperature to fall during the initial stages of exercise. As exercise progresses, the core temperature may rise to 39.6°C. High climatic ambient temperature and insufficient fluid replacement can cause a more serious rise in core temperature, which can result in the following four syndromes of heat-induced injury:

1. *Heat cramp*, which is a form of muscle spasm that can occur in poorly

conditioned athletes following prolonged activity in a hot environment. It is thought that the syndrome is due to hyponatraemia, which may be due either to increased sodium sweat loss or to the dilutional effect of a large fluid replacement.

2. *Heat syncope*, which presents as fainting or light-headedness in an athlete following exercise. It is due to venous pooling in the extremities, with a resultant drop in blood pressure, and usually occurs in an athlete who ceases activity abruptly. First aid measures of elevation of the lower limbs and fluid replacement usually restore the athlete to normal.
3. *Heat exhaustion*, which presents as extreme weakness, excessive sweating, exhaustion, mildly elevated temperature, extreme thirst and reduced urine output. The patient may also present with an alteration in mental state, which can range from anxiety and giddiness to confusion. The treatment of this condition requires rehydration, either orally or intravenously over an hour.
4. *Heat stroke*, which is a medical emergency and indicates the shut down of the thermoregulatory system. The individual presents with psychoneurological disturbance, which may range from confusion to coma, and significant evidence of dehydration. The diagnosis is confirmed by a rectal temperature greater than 40.1°C. Heat stroke requires immediate attention with crash cart support and fluid and electrolyte replacement. Serum sodium in particular has to be monitored, to avoid hypernatraemic cerebral oedema. Prevention of heat stroke can be assisted by scheduling endurance events in humid climates for either early in the morning or after 6 pm in the evening. The environmental heat stress can be predicted by the wet bulb globe temperature (WBGT), which is a temperature humidity and radiation index. If this calculated temperature is above 27.5°C, the event should be rescheduled at a safer time. Below this calculated temperature, a colour coded system can be put into operation to inform the athletes of the climatic conditions.

Further reading: The American College of Sports Medicine (1984). *Position on the Prevention of Thermal Injuries during Distance Running.* The American College of Sports Medicine.

7. Lipids and exercise:

a. False b. False c. False d. False e. True

Regular aerobic exercise is associated with a reduced risk of coronary artery disease. One of the major risk factors for coronary artery disease is an abnormal lipid and lipoprotein profile. Aerobic exercise is associated with an elevation in total high-density lipoprotein HDL2 and in the high-density lipoprotein's major protein component, apoprotein A1. HDL and its subfractions nasant, HDL3 and HDL2 are involved in reverse cholesterol transport from the periphery to the liver, where it is excreted, and are thus associated with an anti-arraetrogenic effect. Low-density lipoprotein (LDL) is positively associated with the development of coronary artery disease. Its major protein is apoprotein B. Aerobic exercise has a variable affect on LDL; research has reported increases, decreases, and no alteration in serum LDL levels following aerobic activity programmes. Lipid profiles can be significantly altered by dietary intake. Higher levels of dietary fibre are associated with a positive lipoprotein profile. Alcohol also alters lipid profiles, and an elevation in high-density lipoprotein has been reported; however, research indicates that the apoprotein A11 (which is not associated with an anti-arraetrogenic action) is elevated, rather than apoprotein A1 (which is considered to be the protective apoprotein).

Further reading: Hughes, V. A., Fiatarone, M. A. and Ferrara, C. M. (1994). Lipoprotein response to exercise training and a low-fat diet in older subjects with glucose intolerance. *Am. J. Clin. Nutr.*, **59**(4), 820–26.

8. Dehydration:

a. True b. False c. False d. False e. False

Dehydration is a constant problem for the athlete who is trying to make weight, and also for athletes exercising in warm climates. Dehydration of the order of 2 per cent of the body weight can significantly reduce aerobic performance. The greater the dehydration, the greater the aerobic performance deficit. Daily weighing in a fit athlete provides an easy method of assessing and replacing fluid loss. A reduction in body weight of 1 kg indicates a fluid deficit of 1 l (a loss of 1 lb indicates a fluid deficit of 1 pint). Dehydration results in decreased blood volume and blood pressure, a reduced blood flow through the kidneys, impaired thermoregulation and a decrease in maximal stroke volume. Under normal circumstances, the body's water content is constant; 60 per cent is derived from our daily water intake, 30 per cent from our food intake and the remaining 10 per cent from the water that is a by-product of oxidated phosphorylation.

Further reading: White, J. A. and Ford, M. A. (1983). The hydration and electrolyte maintenance properties of an experimental sports drink. *Br. J. Sports Med.*, **17**, 51–8.

9. Exercise-induced asthma:

a. True b. False c. False d. True e. True

Increased knowledge of exercise risk factors for development of exercised-induced asthma has led to the suggestion that certain sports are more problematic than others in this regard. High risk sports are those that require continuous exertion at a high percentage of the aerobic capacity, and include cross country snow skiing, ice skating, ice hockey, basketball, soccer, cycling and rowing. Low risk sports are those that require only intermittent exertion at a low percentage of aerobic capacity, and include tennis, volleyball, swimming and gymnastics.

Further reading: Barnes, P. J. (1989). A new approach to the treatment of asthma. *N. Engl. J. Med.*, **321,** 1517-27.

10. Management of exercise-induced asthma:

a. True b. True c. True d. False e. False

Exercise-induced asthma is very common among active people, with an incidence ranging from 3–12 per cent. More than 35 per cent of people who experience allergic rhinitis also experience exercise-induced asthma precipitated by a combination of air pollutants. The overall incidence in the general population is 12–15 per cent. Pulmonary function testing is an integral part of the diagnosis of exercise-induced asthma. Basing the diagnosis of asthma on peak flow values alone may be hazardous, as peak flow readings are highly performance-dependent. A diagnosis of exercise-induced asthma requires FEV1 and FEV1-FEC values below 80 per cent of those predicted. Inhaled corticosteroids form an integral part of the treatment of asthma. Inhaled steroids do not have any immediate bronchodilator effect; however, if they are used on a daily basis they can improve the effectiveness of pre-exercise beta agonists in preventing or decreasing the severity of exercise-induced asthma. Inhaled doses of less then 400 gm per day have a low incidence of side effects. The most common side effects of inhaled steroids are oropharangeal canditis and dysphonia.

Further reading: Mellion, M. B., Kobnegashi, R. H. (1992). Exercise induced asthma. *Am. Fam. Physician*, **45**, 2671-76.

11. Herpes virus infections:

a. False b. True c. True d. True e. True

Herpes viruses can cause a variety of diseases, and include infections due to herpes simplex virus type 1. This infection is commonly seen amongst contact sports participants, and is referred to as 'scrum pox' and 'herpes gladiatorum' among the rugby and wrestling fraternities respectively. Herpes simplex type 1 can cause stomatitis in children, and is associated with cold sores in both young and old. It is associated with erythema multiforme and primary genital herpes in the adult population. Other members of the herpes family include type 2, which mainly causes genital herpes, and varicella-zoster, which is common in the young as chickenpox and in the elderly population as shingles. Rarer human herpes viruses include human herpes 6, which is associated with roseola infantum in children and is suggested to be an aetiological factor in the development of multiple sclerosis. Human herpes virus 7 also causes roseola infantum, but appears to be less pathogenic. Human herpes 8 is strongly associated with Kaposi's sarcoma in AIDS patients.

Further reading: Griffiths, P. D. (1995). Progress in the clinical management of herpes virus infections. *Antiviral Chem. Chemother.*, **6**(4), 191–209.

12. Exercise-induced anaphylaxis:

a. True b. True c. False d. False e. False

Exercise-related allergies vary in severity, from a minor inconvenience and cholinergic urticaria to a life-threatening medical emergency associated with exercise-induced anaphylaxis. Differentiating the two conditions can initially be difficult. Cholinergic urticaria is usually associated with precipitating causes such as exercise, associated emotional stimuli or spicy food; the respiratory symptoms are those of bronchospasm, and the associated rash usually has small weals less than 4 mm in diameter. Anaphylaxis is also caused by exercise and emotional stimuli, and by certain foods such as shellfish. Upper airways obstruction may occur, and the skin rash has giant weals usually greater than 10 mm in diameter. It is almost always associated with pruritus and angio-oedema; flushing is observed in over 75 per cent of cases and syncope and gastrointestinal symptoms can also occur.

Further reading: Terrell, T., Hough, D. O. and Alexander, R. (1996). Identifying exercise allergies. *Phys. Sports Med.*, **24**(11).

13. Sickle-cell trait and sudden death:

a. False b. False c. True d. True e. True

Exertional collapse and sudden death from sickle-cell trait is a particular risk for athletes of African origin, as up to 8 per cent of the African community has sickle-cell trait. The risk of sudden death in these athletes is 1.3 per 1000 for the age group of 23–30 years. It is therefore probably advisable for all athletes from the African continent to be checked for sickle-cell trait during pre-participation screening. Individuals at risk should pay particular attention to their preparation for exercise and should avoid dehydration, which may increase the risk of exertional collapse. Diuretics, antihistamines, caffeine and alcohol should therefore all be avoided prior to engaging in activity. Individuals with sickle-cell trait have a propensity for the red blood cells to form a sickle shape when they are deoxygenated. This can lead to endothenical damage, resulting in vascular occlusion and intervascular coagulation; this is the pathogenesis of collapse and associated death. Individuals who are at risk should be screened for sickle-cell trait prior to engaging in a conditioning programme.

Further reading: Kerle, K. K. and Nishimura, K. D. (1996). Exertional collapse and sudden death associated with sickle-cell trait. *Am. Fam. Physician*, **54**(1), 237–40.

14. Peripheral arterial disease:

a. True b. True c. True d. True e. True

Peripheral arterial disease is a common manifestation of atherosclerosis. It affects about 12 per cent of the general population, and up to 20 per cent of older individuals. Patients with this disease often also have systemic atherosclerosis, and have an increased mortality rate due to cardiovascular diseases. Risk factors for peripheral arterial disease include cigarette smoking, diabetes mellitus, hypertension, hyperlipidaemia, and a reduction in HDL cholesterol. Abnormalities in homocysteine metabolism have also been implicated. Of the major risk factors associated with the development of peripheral arterial disease, only cessation of smoking appears to improve the symptoms of claudication. Intervention therapies include risk factor modification, surgery and angioplasty. Exercise rehabilitation is also a highly effective treatment for claudication, both for peripheral arterial disease and for other cardiovascular pathologies such as coronary artery disease. Walking programmes are associated with an improvement in treadmill exercise performance and in community-based walking ability in persons with claudication symptoms.

Further reading: Criqui, M. H., Fronek, B. and Barrett-Connor, E. (1985). The prevalence of peripheral arterial disease in a defined population. *Circulation*, **71**, 510–15.

15. Hamstrings:

a. False b. False c. False d. False e. False
f. False g. True

Hamstrings take their origin at the ischium and are inserted as the pes anserinas into the medial portion of the tibia just below the joint line. The semimembranosus and semitendinosus receive their nerve supply through the tibial portion of the sciatic nerve, and are predominantly L4, L5 enervated muscles. The biceps femoris has both a long and a short head. The long head is enervated by the tibial portion of the sciatic nerve, and has a predominantly S1, S2 enervation. The short head of the biceps is enervated by the peroneal portion of the sciatic nerve and supplied predominantly from the S1 nerve root. In cases of chronic hamstring injuries an adequate assessment of the lumbosacral spine is required, as lumbosacral disc disease often mimics a chronic hamstring injury.

16. Altitude sickness:

a. False b. True c. True d. False e. False

Acute altitude sickness usually causes the symptoms of dyspnoea, insomnia, headaches and nausea. The insomnia is thought to be associated with the interruption in the normal sleep stages that occurs at altitude. Climbers may also suffer from interrupted or Cheyne–Stokes breathing, which can again interfere with sleep. Acute altitude sickness can be avoided by a gradual ascent, climbing no more than 300 m a day at elevations above

3000 m. High altitude pulmonary oedema is a climbing medical emergency, and occurs most frequently in individuals who rapidly ascend above 2700 m. This condition occurs in otherwise healthy individuals, and appears to be more common in the young. The incidence of HAPO is generally about 50 cases per 100 000 people, but under the age of 14 it is 140 cases per 100 000; this suggests that climbers outgrow the predisposition to developing HAPO as they increase in age. HAPO is treated by administering oxygen and moving the victim to a lower altitude. High altitude cerebral oedema is characterized by confusion progressing to coma and death; most cases are reported at altitudes greater than 4300 m. Treatment is supplementation with oxygen and descent to a lower altitude.

Further reading: Hackett, P. H. and Rennie, D.(1979). The incidence, importance and prophylaxis of acute mountain sickness. *Lancet*, (**ii**), 1449-54.

The team physician

17. Acute management of quadriceps haematoma:

a. True b. True c. True d. True e. False

The acute management of any soft tissue injury can follow the PRICES theorem of first aid:

P – **Protect** the individual from further damaging the injured structure
R – **Rest** the injured structure
I – **Ice**, or cryotherapy, is a very effective way to provide vasoconstriction during the first 24 hours following an injury. Research has suggested that early cryotherapy speeds return to activity. It is important, however, that the ice is not applied directly to the skin as an ice burn may be inflicted. Ideally, olive oil should be applied to the skin and the ice applied via a polythene bag. The ice should be applied for a maximum of 20–25 minutes. The cryotherapy also has the advantage of providing significant analgesia by cooling the sensory nerves and thus reducing sensory nerve conduction.
C – **Compression** is also important in controlling oedema following a muscle injury. Compression may be applied by the application of a crepe bandage or a by more sophisticated intermittent compression system; these systems are now available in combination with cryotemperature systems so that sequential pressure and cooling can be combined.
E – **Elevation** is also important in preventing the accumulation of dependent oedema. The injured subject should be encouraged to either elevate the injured structure or to move it, which will alleviate the tendency to oedema formation to some degree.
S – **Support** the injured structure, either with simple crepe bandage to prevent further bleeding, or in a pressure cuffed device. The athlete must also be supported psychologically, particularly in the first hour following an injury.

Non-steroidal anti-inflammatories are also widely used in the first 24 hours following a musculoskeletal injury. There is some evidence that the non-steroidal anti-inflammatories may adversely affect healing in ligaments and tendons by predisposing to the formation of weaker collagen. However, each case should be judged on its own merits, and frequently the early use of non-steroidals will allow earlier mobilization and recovery.

Further reading: Hocutt, J. E., Jaffe, R. and Rylander, C. R. (1982). Cryotherapy in ankle sprains. *Am. J. Sports Med.*, **10**, 316-19.

18. Delayed onset muscle soreness:

a. True b. True c. True d. False e. True

Muscle soreness that occurs a day or two after heavy exercise is a phenomenon well known to the exerciser, and is referred to as delayed onset muscle soreness (DOMS). The actual pathogenesis of this condition is not yet established, although many theories exist. It is most common following eccentric activity rather than static or concentric actions. Unaccustomed physical activity or a sudden increase in the intensity of activity is commonly associated with this problem. The coexistence of a viral infection has also been cited as a potential cause. The pain can range from mild discomfort to a disabling pain that may require rest and non-steroidal anti-inflammatory medication. There is generalized tenderness affecting a large muscle group, which usually presents 12–48 hours after activity. There is usually no local swelling or bruising, which helps to distinguish it from an acute muscle tear. In severe cases, muscle enzymes may be raised and the muscle cells break down, rarely resulting in myoglobinuria. Warm-down exercises and graded stretching are usually sufficient to treat the discomfort. Prevention is best achieved by grading the workouts to build up gradually over a period of 6–8 weeks.

Further reading: Tiidus, P. M. and Ianuzzo, C. D. (1983). Effects of intensity and duration of muscular exercise on delayed soreness and serum enzyme activity. *Med. Sci. Sports Exer.*, **15**, 461-65.

19. The female athletic triad:

a. False b. False c. True d. False e. True

The young female athlete who is driven to excel in her sport often wants a thin physique. This desire may result in the female athletic triad, which involves an eating disorder, amenorrhoea and osteoporosis. The eating disorder can involve a spectrum of behaviours, from mildly restricted food intake to anorexia or bulimia nervosa. This disordered eating behaviour is regularly observed in female athletes and dancers. Primary amenorrhoea is often observed in these girls, who may not have begun their menses by the age of 16 years. Secondary amenorrhoea may also be observed in the older athlete. Certain studies have observed that athletes who begin training prior to the menarche experience a delay in the onset of menstruation and have an increased incidence of amenorrhoea compared to those who begin training post-menarche. Further research has observed that a decrease in training intensity, frequency and duration alone may precede the onset of menstruation in dancers with delayed menarche. Osteoporosis in the young female athlete may occur as a result of amenorrhoea and oligomenorrhea, and this may be partially irreversible despite the resumption of menses, oestrogen replacement or calcium supplementation. An increased incidence of stress fractures has been reported in these athletes. Vertebral bone mineral density has been observed to be lower in female athletes with a lifelong history of irregular menstruation. A high index of suspicion is required when treating female athletes, and female athletes who present with stress fractures or menstrual irregularities should be screened for female athlete triad. This is not a self-limiting condition. Food restriction and purging can result not only in menstrual dysfunction and bone loss but also in physiological and mental complications. In non-athletic individuals with eating disorders, death rates of as high as 18 per cent have been reported.

Further reading: Daniel, W. A. and Paulshock, B. Z. (1979). A physician's guide to sexual maturity. *Patient Care*, **30**, 122–9.
Drinkwater, B. L. (1985). Women and exercise, the physiological aspects. *Exer. Sports Sci. Rev.*, **5**, 21–51.

20. Spondylolisthesis:

a. True b. False c. True d. False e. False

In 1853, Kilian first described spondylolysis and spondylolisthesis. Spondylosis is a defect in the neural arch, usually at the paras interarticularis, and spondylolisthesis is the slipping of one vertebra on another. This defect is present in approximately 5 per cent of the general population, but is more common in certain groups – for example, Eskimos are reported to have an incidence as high as 50 per cent. The condition may be traumatic, congenital or degenerative. A large number of patients present with spondylolisthesis in association with activity. There is a high incidence in female gymnasts, high jumpers, hurlers, weight-lifters and American Football linesmen; the injuries either occur traumatically or are already present congenitally but become symptomatic following activity. The majority of the slips occur at the L5, S1 level, and they are graded from 1 to 4. A minimal slip is categorized as grade 1, and a slip of greater than 75 per cent is grade 4. The patient will usually present with dull backache, which worsens on activity and may radiate into the buttocks or along the distribution of the sciatic nerve. Plain radiographs often fail to identify the defect, and an oblique X-ray is always required. The spondylolysis will show a 'Scottie dog' defect on X-ray. This is observed by imagining a Scottie dog on the oblique view, where the superior facet makes the dog's ear, the transverse process the snout, the spinus process a hind leg, and the inferior facet the foreleg. The collar of the dog is the level of the pars interarticularis, which is the usual site of the defect. In spondylolisthesis, the vertebra has slipped and the collar of the Scottie dog will widen. Adolescents with a slip of greater than 25 per cent should avoid contact sports unless they are completely asymptomatic and repeat radiology confirms no further progression. In a similar way, isokinetic dynometry should be avoided if a slip is greater than 25 per cent.

Further reading: McGee, D. J. (1997). *Orthopaedic Physical Assessment* 3rd edn. W. B. Saunders.

21. Whiplash injury:

a. True b. False c. True d. True e. False

Whiplash syndrome refers to a jolting type of injury resulting in a hyperextension–hyperflexion injury to the unprotected cervical spine. It is also referred to as a cantilever injury or an acceleration–deceleration trauma. Whilst a whiplash injury is most frequently seen following a motor vehicle accident in which the victim's stationary vehicle was shunted from the rear, it is also not infrequently encountered among the sporting community. It is seen particularly as an acceleration–deceleration trauma in contact sports such as American football and rugby union. The typical pattern is that the patient complains of general shock and anxiety. Following a variable period of hours or even days, the patient generally presents with aching cervical muscles, headache and tinnitus. Neck pain is almost universal in cases of whiplash; headache is present in upwards of 80 per cent of patients, and is usually dependent on the severity of the injury. Dysphagia and pain in the shoulder, arm, chest and even the lower back are all commonly encountered following a whiplash injury. The whiplash injury can be classified into three groups:

1. Group 1 – symptoms with no objective signs on clinical examination
2. Group 2 – symptoms and limitation of neck movement, but no abnormal neurological signs
3. Group 3 – symptoms, limitation of neck movement, and objective and neurological signs.

Whilst a whiplash injury appears to be a self-limiting condition, it is reported that upwards of 90 per cent of patients continue to have significant symptoms after 2 years. Long-term follow-up radiology also confirms the increased incidence of degenerative spondylosis after whiplash. Typically, the spondylotic changes are confined to one or two segments at the C5, 6 and 7 level. The treatment of whiplash injury is currently largely empirical. In the sports setting there is usually no medico-legal compensation case pending, and symptoms described are therefore rarely other than genuine. Symptomatic treatment is directed towards the specific pathology, and often includes antispasmodic agents, non-steroidal anti-inflammatories, early mobilization, facet joint injections and trigger point injections.

Further reading: Brown, J. N. and Crosby, A. C. (1993). Acute soft tissue injury of the cervical spine. *Br. Med. J.*, **307**, 439–40.

22. Exertional compartment syndrome of the leg:

a. True b. False c. False d. False e. True

Exertional compartment syndrome is most commonly seen in the lower leg, and tends to appear in sedentary people who commence a vigorous programme unsupervised. Chronic compartment syndrome usually affects younger, conditioned athletes. There are four compartments in the lower leg; the anterior and deep posterior compartments are those most often affected in this condition, whereas the lateral and superficial posterior compartments are affected much less frequently. Each compartment contains a major nerve and, therefore, neurological symptoms may be a significant presenting feature. The tibial nerve runs through the deep posterior compartment, the deep peroneal nerve through the anterior compartment, the superficial peroneal nerve through the lateral compartment and the sural through the superficial posterior compartment. The history is usually that of pain, swelling and paraesthesiae following activity. The diagnosis of compartment syndrome can be made using pressure studies, which will observe an abnormal increase in pressure during and following activity. It is suggested that resting pressure studies above 15 mmHg and 20 mmHg post-exercise are diagnostic of compartment syndrome. X-rays are usually normal, and bone scanning may be performed to rule out a local stress fracture. MRI scanning is occasionally used to identify muscle abnormalities.

Further reading: Edwards, P. and Myerson, M. S. (1996). Exertional compartment syndrome of the leg. *Phys. Sports Med.*, **24**(4).

23. Emotional stress:

a. True b. False c. False d. True e. True

Competition regularly increases the emotional strain on sportsmen and women. This may be manifested by behavioural changes such as hand tremor, agitation and aggressiveness, or by physiological changes such as alterations in muscle tone, blood pressure, heart rate and urine and blood contents. Elevated pre-competition heart rates have been observed by various investigators in a variety of sports; in particular, participants in stressful activities such as motor racing and downhill skiing have significantly raised pre-competition heart rates. American football, soccer and wrestling, on the other hand, have only modest elevations in pre-competition heart rates. The heightened psychological state has been associated with an increase in the incidence of injury, which suggests that the psychological reactions are increased beyond an optimal level. A variety of athletes may suffer from pre-competition stress; however, research has indicated that individuals holding the more responsible positions (such as goalkeeper) show the greatest stress, and that stress-related pathologies peak during the more important parts of the sports season. These psychological stresses have also been shown to alter the size of the thyroid gland over a short period of heightened activity.

Further reading: Reilly, T. (1997). Pre-start moods of cross-country runners and the relationship to performance. *Int. J. Sports Psychol.*, **8**, 210–17.

24. Swimmer's shoulder:

a. True b. False c. True d. False e. True

Shoulder pain caused by impingement of the subacromial tissues is a common overuse injury seen in the swimming fraternity. This was first described as swimmer's shoulder in 1974. It most commonly occurs with freestyle and butterfly strokes, and has been reported to affect up to 75 per cent of all competitive swimmers. The pain in swimmer's shoulder occurs due to repeated extreme adduction and abduction, which compresses the soft tissue in the subacromial space between the head of the humerus and the coraco-acromial arch. These structures are put under particular stress during the freestyle stroke adduction and internal rotation during the early and mid pull-through phase, and during extreme abduction during the recovery phase of the swimming stroke. Swimmer's shoulder is an overuse injury and, as with all overuse injuries, relative rest and activity modification is the mainstay of treatment. Treatment also includes the specific treatment of inflammation, and correction of any muscle imbalance in the rotator cuff and scapula stabilizers to ensure restoration of normal gleno-humeral stability. Rehabilitation of the parascapula muscles can often be difficult; however, protracted push-ups have been shown to improve the function of the rhomboid minor and rhomboid major.

Further reading: Kennedy, J. C. and Hawkins, R. J. (1974). Swimmer's shoulder. *Phys. Sports Med.*, **2**(4), 34–8.

25. Wet bulb temperature:

a. True b. True c. True d. True e. True

The wet bulb temperature provides the simplest assessment of environmental heat stress. The wet bulb temperature is obtained by first wetting a wick wrapped around a bulb of a thermometer, and then determining the effective evaporation of moisture from the wick at the thermometer's temperature. This thermometer is referred to as a wet bulb thermometer. A wet bulb thermometer and a dry bulb thermometer are combined together in the sling psychometer, which is used to produce evaporation. The wet bulb temperature never exceeds the dry bulb temperature. When they are equal, the air is completely saturated with water vapour and the relative humidity is 100 per cent; therefore, no further evaporation is possible. The amount of evaporation depends upon wind currents and on the quantity of water in the air. The sling psychometer can be used to assess environmental heat stress; by containing both a dry bulb and a wet bulb thermometer, the temperature and the relative humidity of the air can be measured. A wet bulb temperature index has been suggested that gives a guide to the degree of environmental stress on athletes.

Further reading: Murphy, R. J. and Ashe, W. F. (1965). Prevention of heat illness in football players. *JAMA*, **194**(6), 650–54.

26. Nasal injury:

a. True b. True c. True d. True e. False

Nasal injuries are very commonly encountered in sports. The nose is one of the areas most frequently fractured among the sporting community. Injuries are often due to fighting in contact sports such as rugby and ice hockey; direct blows in racket sports can also occur accidentally, and collisions whilst heading a soccer ball or rising to catch a Gaelic football are other causes. Protective facial equipment, such as hurling helmets, has reduced the overall incidence of nasal injuries. Nasal contusions can result in septal haematomas, which may ultimately cause cartilage damage due to necrobiosis, and careful examination is therefore essential following these injuries so the haematoma may be drained if necessary in order to avoid this outcome. Lacerations should also be carefully examined; those involving the nasal cartilage require great care to ensure no cartilage is left exposed. With complicated nasal lacerations, a speedy referral to an ENT or plastic surgeon is essential. Epistaxis is the most commonly encountered nasal injury. Anterior bleeding is usually from the vessels in the anterior septum (Kiesselbach's area), and bleeding from this area is usually well controlled with direct pressure. Posterior bleeding generally drains into the throat, and is usually from the posterior ethmoidal artery; bleeding from this area is controlled by elevation of the head and nasal packing. For uncontrollable bleeding, local pressure such as an internal balloon may be necessary prior to specialist referral.

Further reading: Schendel, S. A. (1990). Sports related nasal injuries. *Phys. Sports Med.*, **18** (10), 59.

27. Elbow pain in the tennis-playing population:

a. False b. False c. True d. True e. False

Classic 'tennis elbow' refers only to lateral elbow symptoms, and 75 per cent of 'tennis elbows' are localized at the lateral epicondyle at the attachment of the common extensor muscles. Seventeen per cent of the symptoms are localized to the lateral muscle mass at the musculo-tendinous junction of the common extensor muscles, which is proximal to the radial head; 10 per cent are on the medial aspect at a level of the medial epicondyle, where the common flexor origin attaches to the humerus; and 8 per cent occur posteriorly around the margins of the olecranon process. The total of site adds up to greater than 100 per cent because individuals may experience pain at more than one site.

On rare occasions the posterior interosseous nerve may be the cause of lateral elbow pain in tennis players, and also in those who perform a repetitive task with their forearm. This is caused by entrapment of the nerve as it traverses the supinator muscle, and it usually results in weakness and pain in the extensor muscle complex. EMG evaluation usually shows sparing of the radial nerve-innervated brachioradialis and extensor carpi-radialis and supinator muscles. However, distal extensor muscles and the abductor policis longus, which are supplied by the posterior interosseous nerve, are usually affected, and show evidence of denervation.

Further reading: Leach, R. E. and Miller, J. K. (1987). Lateral and medial epicondylitis of the elbow. *Clin. Sports Med.*, **6**(2), 259-72.

28. Sports brassieres:

a. False   b. False   c. False   d. True   e. False

Breast injury is a female-specific sports injury, although jogger's nipple can occur in both males and females. This is a painful chapping of the nipple caused by friction, and can be avoided by placing tape over the nipple and aureole before exercise. Excessive breast motion during exercise can cause sagging and local trauma, and a properly fitting bra can support the breasts and avoid these consequences. The fabric of the bra should be non-allergic, absorbent and, ideally, at least 50 per cent cotton to allow ventilation and decrease chafing. The straps should be wide for comfort. Elasticated fabric, however, should be avoided, as its movement will lead to further chafing. The seams should also avoid the nipple line, as this will cause further irritation. It is suggested that women with B cup sizes or less should use a compressing or binding brassiere, whilst a firmer encapsulating support bra is suggested for women with C cup sizes or larger. In the latter garment, each breast is held in its own cup.

Further reading: Lyle, J. M. and Micheli, L. (1995). Sports medicine concerns of female athletes. In *The Sports Medicine Bible*. Harper Collins.

29. Biomechanical abnormalities:

a. True   b. False   c. False   d. True   e. True

Biomechanical abnormalities may predispose an athlete to a combination of overuse injuries. Everyday walking and activities are generally insufficient to provoke an overuse injury; however, injuries may occur when the limb is subjected to repetitive and repeated stress. Common lower limb biomechanical abnormalities include pes planus (flat feet). A flattened medial arch may result in excessive pronation and, as a result, the lower limb is susceptible to injury. A trochanteric bursitis at the hip, patello-femoral syndrome at the knee joint and compartment syndrome of the lower leg can all be attributed to pes planus and hyperpronation. Foot problems include stress fractures and posterior tibial tendonitis. Pes cavus (high arch of the foot) is associated with a rigid foot; the shock-absorbing ability of the foot is therefore decreased, and stresses associated with activity are transmitted to the lower limb. Therefore, athletes with pes cavus are susceptible to stress fractures throughout the lower limb. Plantar fasciitis and Achilles tendonitis are also both common owing to the poor shock-absorbing ability of the foot. Hammer toes and metatarsalgias can develop due to the excessive forces placed on the forefoot. Genu valgum (knocked knees) is a cause of patellofemoral syndrome due to the inward turn of the kneecap, resulting in maltracking at the patellofemoral joint. In a similar way, femoral anteversion also causes maltracking problems for the kneecap, which also faces inwards and leaves the individual susceptible to patellofemoral syndrome. Genu varum (bow legs) results in angulation of the knees outwards. This biomechanical abnormality can increase the likelihood of the ilio-tibial band friction syndrome. This is caused by excessive stretching of the band across the knee joint, and may result in a secondary condition of trochanteric bursitis. The patient may present with symptoms of trochanteric bursitis, with localized pain on hip abduction. Careful biomechanical assessment may identify genu varum, which may be the precipitating cause of the ilio-tibial band friction syndrome and secondary trochanteric bursitis.

30. Tineanea cruris:

a. False b. False c. False d. True e. False

Tineanea cruris is more commonly known as 'jock itch'. It is a common complaint among male athletes, and rarely affects females. Symptoms include red, scaly, itchy patches on the groin, thighs and buttocks. Occasionally there may be an associated secondary bacterial infection. Poor hygiene, inadequate ventilation of the groin area and friction are the primary causes of this condition, and it is therefore common among obese athletes or in those with heavily muscled thighs that rub together during exercise. Tight-fitting athletic apparel is also a contributory factor, and ill-fitting athletic supports or those made of synthetic material can contribute to the condition. Treatment involves careful attention to hygiene and, in particular, avoiding standing around in damp or sweaty athletic apparel after exercise. Anti-fungal agents are often prescribed by the physician to speed up resolution of the condition.

31. Rhabdomyolysis:

a. True b. True c. True d. False e. True

Rhabdomyolysis is a rare condition. It can occur in association with exercise and a variety of other unrelated pathologies. Signs and symptoms of rhabdomyolysis include diffuse muscle pain, muscle swelling, hyperkalaemia, hyperphosphataemia and hypo-uricaemia. The patient's urine will be red and the urinalysis will test positive for haem. Muscle enzymes are also elevated (creatine, lactate dehydrogenase and serum glutamic-oxaloacetic transaminase). The exercise-related rhabdomyolysis is usually associated with severe muscle activity and has also been associated with a sudden excessive increase in activity or if exercise takes place in association with a viral or bacterial infection. The rhabdomyolysis can rapidly lead to acute renal failure, and this is therefore the cardinal element to treat in cases of rhabdomyolysis. Intravenous fluid and bicarbonate and mannitol infusions to maintain a urine pH at greater than 6.5 can be effective. Rhabdomyolysis has been reported among military recruits who engage in vigorous activity during hot weather. It has also been reported in poorly conditioned athletes taking activity during hot weather. In these instances it can be associated with disseminated intervascular coagulation.

Further reading: Better, O. S. and Stein, J. H. (1990). Early management of shock and prophylaxis of acute renal failure in traumatic rhabdomyolysis. *N. Engl. J. Med.*, **322**(12), 825–9.

32. Injuries to the male genito-urinary system:

a. True b. True c. True d. False e. True

The male genitalia are rarely injured during athletic activity. Injury is usually caused by a local trauma, and the wearing of athletic supports to elevate the testes protects individuals in susceptible sports – such as baseball catchers, hockey players and cricketers. Sexually transmitted diseases are the most common urological problem of the male athlete. Non-gonococcal urethritis is the most commonly encountered condition, and patients will present with urethral discharge and dysuria. Chlamydial infections are a common offender, and usually respond to a 7-day course of tetracycline. The sports medicine physician will regularly be consulted regarding scrotal masses. Testicular cancer is the most common malignancy in the 16–35-year-old male; therefore, the presence of a mass in the testes separate from the epididymis must initially be considered malignant, and requires prompt investigation. A mass separate from the testes should be evaluated by transillumination with a bright light. Hydroceles will transilluminate; however, a mass will not. Varicoceles may be present in up to 19 per cent of all males. These are varicosities of the internal spermatic vein, and are often described as a 'bag of worms'. In the absence of symptoms, these varicoceles often do not require any further management.

Further reading: York, P. J. (1990). Sport and the male genito-urinary system. *Phys. Sports Med.*, **18**(10).

33. Heat cramps:

a. True b. False c. False d. True e. False

Heat illness is a spectrum of conditions ranging from the mild symptoms of heat cramps to the medical emergency of heat stroke. Heat cramps usually occur in the calf muscle following strenuous or prolonged activity. The core temperature is usually normal, but may be elevated as high as 38.5°C. The calf muscles are most susceptible; however, any muscle can be affected and the abdominal muscles, if affected, may mimic an acute appendix. Hyponatraemia or poor hydration increases the likelihood of heat cramps. If an athlete presents with heat cramps, treatment is by resting in a cool place and rehydration. If heat cramps occur in children, it may take a number of hours for full hydration to occur and, therefore, activity may be terminated for the day. Children who are at particular risk of heat illness include those who are obese or poorly conditioned; children with cystic fibrosis, diabetes mellitus and congenital heart disease are also more susceptible to heat-related illness.

Further reading: Gutierrez, G. and Tanner, S. M. (1995). Solar injury and heat illness. *Phys. Sports Med.*, **23**(7).

34. Osgood–Schlatter's disease:

a. True b. True c. True d. False e. False

Osgood–Schlatter's disease is commonly encountered in the active adolescent. It is usually a self-limiting condition, and affects the tibial tuberosity. The X-ray findings show loss of homogeneity of the infrapatellar fat pad. There can also be obliteration of the inferior angle of the fat pad, irregularity and thickening of the tissues between the anterior surface of the tibia and the posterior margin of the fat pad. Patellar tendon thickening is also regularly observed on lateral X-rays. Fragmentation of the tibial tuberosity is the most obvious finding; however, it is also the most variable. The tibial tuberosity is lateral to the midline of the tibia and, therefore, lateral X-rays with the tibia in slight internal rotation are recommended.

Further reading: Woolfrey, B. F. and Chandler, E. F. (1960). Manifestations of Osgood–Schlatter's disease in the late teens and early adulthood. *J. Bone Joint Surg.*, **42A**(2), 327–32; 369.

35. Sinding-Larsen–Johansson disease:

a. False b. True c. False d. False e. True

In 1920, Sinding-Larsen and Johansson independently described a syndrome affecting athletic adolescents. The condition usually affects children between the age of 10 and 13 years. Pain may be caused by running, kneeling and ascending stairs. There is usually tenderness at the inferior pole of the patella, and this can be exacerbated by resisted quadriceps contractions. The condition is associated with other adolescent overuse syndromes such as Osgood–Schlatter's disease and Sever's disease. Present thinking considers this condition to be due to necrosis of the tendon fibres, with secondary calcification at the inferior pole of the patella. A further hypothesis is that of local patellar avulsion, with resultant ossification. It is usually due to repetitive traction of the patella tendon at the patella, and is regularly seen in adolescents who are athletic; it can also be seen in children who enjoy playing on bouncy castles. The calcification near the inferior pole of the patella can occur within weeks of the onset of the acute symptoms. X-ray appearances can range from normal irregular calcification at the inferior pole of the patella to incorporation of the calcification within the patella, which often yields a normal appearance on lateral X-rays. Activity modification is the keystone to recovery; occasionally, plaster cast immobilization is required. In the natural course of the condition, it may be up to 1 year before the patient becomes pain free. It does not usually require surgical intervention, and most children continue to have active teenage years.

Further reading: Sinding-Larsen, M. F. (1921) A hitherto unknown affliction of the patella in children. *Acta Radiol.*, **1**, 171–3.

36. Tietze's syndrome:

a. True b. False c. False d. True e. False

Tietze's syndrome is a rare anterior chest wall condition that is regularly confused with costochondritis. It is described as a painful, non-suppurative swelling of the cartilage at its articulation. Tietze's syndrome usually affects young males and females. The actual cause is unknown; a traumatic pathogenesis has been suggested. It presents with swelling and inflammatory changes at the costo-cartilage, and it is more common in the upper ribs, particularly the second and third. It usually affects only one level. The sternoclavicular and xiphisternal articulations may sometimes be involved. It is occasionally associated with respiratory tract infections, and the anterior chest pain is made worse by coughing. This condition has to be differentiated from costochondritis, which occurs at all ages and usually affects a number of rib levels, in particular the second to the sixth. Costochondritis is associated with trauma and fibrositis syndrome. The condition is usually self-limiting, and runs a relapsing course over 1–4 months. Treatment is directed towards the symptoms of pain.

Further reading: Dunlop, R. F. (1969). Tietze's revisited. *Clin. Orthopaed.*, **62**, 223.

Sports injuries

37. Iliac crest apophysitis:

a. False b. True c. False d. True e. True

The iliac crest is the site of attachment of numerous muscles. The gluteus maximus and fibres of the latissimus dorsi muscles attach to the posterior aspect of the iliac crest, and the tensor fascialata, gluteus medius, transverse abdominus and internal and external oblique abdominal muscles attach to the anterior iliac spine. An iliac crest apophysitis is thought to be caused by the reaction of the unfused apophysis to repetitive musculature contraction, or by a subclinical stress fracture of the apophysis. The patient usually presents with a gradual onset of hip pain, localized to the anterior iliac crest, while running. There is usually no history of sudden onset of pain (which would be the case with an acute avulsion fracture). There is usually local tenderness at the anterior iliac crest, and resisted hip abduction may increase pain; however, the range of movement of the hip will be full. X-rays are usually normal, but can show some widening of the iliac apophysis. A bone scan may show increased uptake at the iliac crest on the blood pool and delayed images, and can be helpful in excluding a local avulsion injury. Conservative treatment usually ensures a return to activity in 6 weeks.

Further reading: Paletta, G. A. and Andrish, J. T. (1995). Injuries about the hip and pelvis in the young athlete. *Clin. Sports Med.*, **14**(3), 591-628.

38. Posterior interosseous neuropathy:

a. True b. False c. True d. True e. False

The posterior interosseous nerve (PIN) is a motor branch of the radial nerve. It is most vulnerable to entrapment at the level of the supinator muscle. It is a purely motor nerve, which innervates the majority of the extensors of the forearm. Many patients with PIN entrapment syndrome engage in repetitive forearm rotation or hyperextension activities. In a review of PIN syndrome, over 82 per cent of patients had jobs requiring repetitive movements. This syndrome frequently mimics lateral epicondylitis, as there is often discomfort in the extensor apparatus of the forearm and weakness of the forearm extensor muscles.

The diagnosis of PIN syndrome is usually made electrodiagnostically.

The radially innervated muscles above the site of entrapment are usually spared (extensor carpi radialis and longus, brevis and supinator), and the muscles below the site of entrapment show evidence of denervation (extensor carpi ulnaris, extensor indicis proprius and extensor digitorum communis). The condition is usually painful, and avoidance of the provoking stimulus is the mainstay of treatment. Splinting to reduce rotatory and hyperextension motion can also be used.

Further reading: Lutz, F. R. (1991). Radial tunnel syndrome. An etiology of chronic lateral elbow pain. *J. Orthopaed. Sports Phys. Ther.*, 14(1), 14-17.

39. Lower limb athletic neuropathy:

a. True b. False c. False d. True e. False

Neuropathies comprise a relatively small yet clinically significant subset of athletic injuries. In a large study of peripheral nerve injuries, 5.7 per cent were sports related. Peroneal neuropathy is the most frequently encountered lower limb nerve injury among athletes. Football players and martial arts athletes may sustain direct peroneal nerve injury at the fibular head due to an errant kick, and runners who develop an acute or chronic compartment syndrome may have an accompanying peroneal neuropathy. This nerve is also vulnerable following knee surgery.

Rare neuropathies can be associated with particular athletic activities. Lateral femoral cutaneous neuropathy can occur in a number of sports, and is often referred to as meralgia paraesthetica. It is reported in gymnasts, who may injure the nerve due to impact on the parallel bars, and also in weight-lifters, due to the wearing of tight belts and trusses.

The saphenous nerve, which is the large cutaneous branch of the femoral nerve, supplies sensation to the antero-medial surface of the knee and calf. It can be injured in a variety of locations along its course. Injuries in Hunter's canal have been reported in running and skiing, and at the level of the pes anserinus following knee injury. Injuries have also been reported in surfers, on the medial aspect of the knee where the nerve becomes subcutaneous. It is suggested that this latter injury occurs while the surfer straddles the surf board waiting for a wave.

Sciatic neuropathy is also a rare cause of sports-related neuropathy. The majority of these entrapments occur in the buttock area or proximal thigh. Entrapment of the sciatic nerve by the piriformis muscle has caused much debate over many years. It is suggested that it occurs in runners and gymnasts, and requires a very specific criteria for diagnosis. A full-blown syndrome is rarely seen.

Sural neuropathy can occur in the popliteal fossa as a complication of knee surgery, and has also been reported after wearing ski boots. The patient complains of an altered sensation along the lateral border of the foot.

40. Ulnar collateral ligament injury (skier's thumb):

a. True b. True c. True d. True e. False

The ulnar collateral ligament stabilizes the metacarpo-phalangeal joint at the base of the thumb. Injury to this structure is usually caused by a forced abduction injury to the thumb. It is frequently seen in skiers, and usually occurs when falling with the ski pole in the hand. Skier's thumb provides 60 per cent of all upper limb problems associated with skiing, and the condition frequently goes undiagnosed. On clinical examination, there is swelling and tenderness on the medial side of the metacarpo-phalangeal joint. The key pinch grip becomes weak due to ligament disruption. A valgus stress is applied in abduction to the thumb in both a flexed and an extended position. Normally, the range of movement is up to 20° in men and 25° in women. If a valgus stress allows an instability of more than 35°, then a ligament rupture is likely. Radiology is essential to clarify whether there are any bony fragments present, and will also identify a Grade 1, 2, or 3 tear. The more significant Grade 3 (Sterner lesion) tear will always require a surgical repair, this may involve pin fixation and open reduction.

Further reading: Ferber, C., Senne, E., Matter, P. (1981). Skier's thumb. *Am. J. Sports Med.*, **9**(3), 171-7.

41. Ulnar nerve palsy:

a. True b. False c. False d. False e. False

An ulnar nerve palsy is quite commonly reported in cyclists and baseball catchers. The site of injury is usually Guyon's canal. This canal is on the hypothenar side of the wrist, and is formed by the hamate and pisiform bones. The ulnar nerve and artery traverse the canal before supplying the hand. The injury in cyclists is usually caused by direct pressure on the nerve from the handlebars. The patient frequently presents with altered sensation in the area of the little finger progressing to weakness of the hypothenar and interosseous muscles of the hand, which are innervated by the ulnar nerve. Not all the sensory divisions of the ulnar nerve are affected, as the dorsal cutaneous nerve (which supplies the dorsum of the hand) separates in the forearm and does not traverse Guyon's canal. This condition has been reported for many years, and is frequently seen in Tour de France cyclists. Changing the grip from the top of the handlebars to the side and the use of padding is often sufficient to prevent the ulnar nerve palsy from deteriorating. Should the symptoms persist, further investigation of the cervical spine should be undertaken to rule out a radiculopathy.

Further reading: Frontera, W. R. (1983). Cyclist's palsy: clinical and electrodiagnostic findings. *Br. J. Sports Med.*, **17**(2), 91–3.

42. Keinbock's disease:

a. False b. True c. True d. False e. False

Avascular necrosis of the lunate bone was first described in 1910 by Robert Keinbock. It usually affects men between the ages of 18 and 40 years, and over 95 per cent of sufferers engage in manual work using their upper limbs. It occurs in athletes who repeatedly use their wrist joint, such as rowers. The cause of this condition is unknown, but it is postulated that it may begin with repeated overuse of the wrist, which results in fracture, or a ligament injury, which results in wrist degeneration. It is also suggested that the interruption in blood supply to the lunate bone may be caused by a primary circulatory problem. Abnormalities of the ulnar bone where it can be seen to lie more proximal than the radial head on postero-anterior X-ray (negative ulnar variance) may predispose to Kienbock's disease. The injury has to be differentiated from carpal fractures, tumours, soft tissue injuries and nerve entrapment around the wrist. The diagnosis is confirmed by X-ray, which will show increased lunate density and flattening. These plain X-rays may be normal in early cases of Kienbock's disease, and MRI scanning is then required to establish the diagnosis, as it can identify the loss of bone marrow fat. Immobilization is the usual early treatment of this condition; however, the results are unsatisfactory, and surgery involving ulnar lengthening, radial shortening and a variety of carpal bone fusions is usually employed.

43. Osteitis pubis:

a. False b. True c. True d. False e. False

Osteitis pubis is an injury of the groin that has been described as an erosion of the pubic symphysis, which is caused by overuse and overload of hip adductors and internal thigh rotators. This condition is common in sports involving unilateral leg support, such as kicking sports, and in activities that involve 'zig-zagging'. It is particularly common in midfield players in soccer and hockey, and in rugby half-backs. The patient may present with an acute or chronic unilateral or bilateral groin pain; it is usually relieved by rest and exacerbated by activity. The pain may radiate into the hip, genitalia or abdomen. Clinically, there is pain at the pubic symphysis, and groin pain on compression of the iliac crests. There is usually no tenderness at the external ring, which is pathognomonic of a Gilmore's groin. The patient usually has limitation of hip adduction and abduction secondarily to local muscle spasm. Hip X-rays may show a variety of abnormalities; irregularity of the periosteum of the pubic bone with bone resorption at the medial ends of the pubic rami, sclerosis of the pubic symphysis and widening of the symphysis. This may be evaluated further by flamingo (alternate single leg standing) views. Three-phase bone scanning is helpful in confirming the diagnosis. However, a positive scan with negative plain X-rays suggests a pubic symphysitis, which is a precursor to osteitis pubis or a stress fracture. Conservative treatment, including supervised rest, NSAIDs and local steroid injection, are advocated in the early stages. Many cases will resolve spontaneously. It is essential to rehabilitate the hip adductors and thigh internal rotators adequately before recommencing full activity. Full recovery can be expected in 7–9 months.

Further reading: Fricker, P. A., Taunton, J. E. and Ammann, W. (1991). Osteitis pubis in athletes: infection, inflammation or injury? *Sports Med.*, **12**(4), 266–79.

44. Plantar fasciitis:

a. False b. False c. False d. True e. True

Plantar fasciitis usually presents as a local point of tenderness at the calcaneus, and occurs especially along the medial tubercle. The point of tenderness is usually acute on first rising in the morning. Plantar fasciitis is most commonly seen in runners who cover 30 miles or more weekly. Predisposing factors include poorly fitting shoes; tight Achilles tendon; poor great toe motion and plantar flexion of 60° or more during the runner's gait. The condition is sometimes relieved with activity, but returns at rest. X-rays often show a traction spur of the calcaneus. This is usually a secondary finding, and is not the cause of the local pain. Treatment includes local shock-absorbing orthotics, gastrocnemius stretching, anti-inflammatories, steroid injection and reduction in weight-bearing activities. Occasionally, surgery is required.

Further reading: Taunton, J. E., Clement, D. B. and McNicol, K. (1982). Plantar fasciitis in runners. *Can. J. Appl. Sports* Sci., **7**(1), 41-4.

45. Osgood–Schlatter's disease:

a. False b.True c. False d. True e. True

Osgood–Schlatter's disease is a painful enlargement of the tibial tuberosity at the patellar tendon insertion. It is an overuse injury that is commonly seen in pre-adolescent and early adolescent children, and usually occurs during a rapid growth period. The condition is caused by repetitive stress on the growing tibial tuberosity apophysis. Pre-disposing factors include abnormality of the patella, such as patella alta or bejon, and muscle imbalance between the quadriceps and hamstring complexes. Clinical examination reveals local tenderness at the tibial tuberosity and, occasionally, tight muscular structures about the knee joint. Radiology is performed to rule out avulsion fractures or malignancies of the tibial tuberosity. Treatment is usually that of activity modification. This is generally a self-limiting condition that resolves spontaneously at the age of 15 or 16 years.

46. Olecranon impingement syndrome:

a. True b. True c. True d. True e. True

Olecranon impingement syndrome is often called 'boxer's elbow'. It is an overuse injury caused by repetitive valgus extension of the elbow, which results in the olecranon process being forced against the medial side of the olecranon fossa. The elbow pain usually develops insidiously, and is experienced on elbow extension. Clinically, there is posterior elbow pain and pain on forced extension with valgus stress. Radiology may show evidence of hypertrophy of the olecranon, spurring of the olecranon tip and, occasionally, loose bodies at the posterior elbow. Conservative measures are first used to treat this painful condition, and alteration in throwing and boxing mechanics are also indicated. Occasionally, removal of the olecranon tip or loose bodies may be required.

47. Burner syndrome (brachial plexus injury):

a. True b. False c. False d. True e. False

Burner (or stinger) syndrome is a very frequently encountered contact sport injury. It is particularly common in American football, with an incidence of up to 65 per cent reported. It is also seen in rugby players, wrestlers, hockey players and gymnasts, and in association with motor vehicle injuries. A burner syndrome involves trauma to the brachial plexus; the injury can be a traction or compression injury of the plexus, a root lesion, or a combination of all aetiologies. The most common mechanism reported is that of traction and stretching of the brachial plexus, causing a downward force on the shoulder and an extension force on the neck, and resulting in a traction injury to the upper trunk of the brachial plexus. Burner syndrome can be divided into three grades. Grade 1, the mildest lesion, is a neurapraxia, which usually recovers within a few days. Grade 2 produces motor and sensory deficits, and can last for up to 2 weeks. Electromyographic evaluation shows evidence of acute denervation, with abnormalities of insertional activity. These findings are only visible 3 weeks after injury. Grade 3 burners are neurotmesis; these injuries have a poor prognosis, and motor and sensory deficits may last indefinitely. Electromyographic changes show evidence of chronic denervation with large polyphasic units on recruitment. There may be no evidence of abnormality in insertional activity. The mainstay of initial diagnosis of a brachial plexus injury is that of the clinical examination. The upper trunk is most commonly affected, and the supraspinatus, biceps and deltoid are therefore frequently involved and will show evidence of motor weakness on resisted testing. The initial treatment of burner syndrome involves general first aid to the affected muscles; this can include the PRICES method of soft tissue first aid (see Answer 17). Following the initial first aid, rehabilitation is commenced. Initially, full range of shoulder movement is obtained, followed by isometric strengthening. This should concentrate on shoulder abduction, internal and external rotation and paraspinal muscle strengthening. If neurogenic muscle weakness has occurred, strength training should be avoided as this may damage motor end plates. In these cases, evidence of electromyographic renervation, such as satellite potentials and large polyphasic units, must be observed prior to commencing resistance rehabilitation.

Further reading: Clancy, W. G. Jnr., Brand, R. L. and Bergfield, J. A. (1977). Upper trunk brachial plexus injuries in contact sports. *Am. J. Sports Med.*, **5**(5), 209–16.

48. Blow-out fractures of the orbit:

a. True b. False c. True d. False e. True

Blow-out fractures of the orbit usually occur following a direct blow to the eye from a fist, knee or blunt object. The thin inferior and medial margins of the orbit are the most frequently damaged. Detection of an orbital fracture can be difficult due to the overlapping contours of the normal lower orbital margin, which consists of the anterior inferior rim of the orbit and the deeper-seated posterior lowermost bony margin of the orbit. In the case of a fracture of the orbital floor, a third line may be present, which indicates a lose bony fragment. However, this is not always present, and more often the only radiological abnormality will be a downward bulging of the peri-orbital soft tissue. This will alter the upper maxillary sinus margin. Due to the abnormal connection between the sinus and the orbit, blowing against the closed glottis will increase the intraorbital pressure and may be the first clinical hint that there is a blow-out fracture of the orbital floor.

Further reading: Fueger, G. F., Milauskas, A. T. and Britton, W. (1966). The Roentgenologic evaluation of orbital blow-out injuries. *J. Roentgenol.*, **97**, 614–17.

49. Malignant brain oedema syndrome:

a. False b. True c. True d. False e. False

The malignant brain oedema syndrome is found in paediatric athletes. It consists of rapid neurological deterioration from a conscious state to coma and occasional death; this occurs following trauma to the head. Autopsy investigation shows a diffuse swelling of the brain with a little or no injury. The cerebral swelling is a result of vascular engorgement. The fatal neurological outcome is usually secondary to raised intracranial pressure. Therefore, early recognition assists prompt treatment with osmotic agents, incubation and hyperventilation to avoid a fatal outcome.

Further reading: Bruce, D. A., Schut, L. and Bruno, L. A. (1978). Outcome following severe head injuries in children. *J. Neurosurg.*, **48**, 679–88.

Musculoskeletal medicine

50. Q angle:

a. True b. False c. False d. True e. True

The quadriceps (Q) angle is measured when the quadriceps is contracted. It is the angle between a line drawn from the anterior superior iliac spine to the midpoint of the patella, and a line from the midpoint of the patella to the tibial tuberosity. The normal Q angle in males is 10° or less. The normal Q angle in females is 16° or less. An increased Q angle is one of the anatomical factors that may contribute to patellofemoral stress syndromes and patellar subluxation. Excessive internal rotation of the hip produces overpronation of the foot at the midstance stage of the running gait. This creates a marked increase of the functional Q angle at the knee, and this is thought to increase loading on the patellofemoral joint with resultant injury in youngsters. Excessive Q angles are frequently found in individuals who have non-traumatic patellar dislocations.

There is much variation in the reporting of normal values for Q angles. It is therefore important to conform to an exact measurement procedure, as small errors in marking the bony structures (anterior superior iliac spine, central and tibial tuberosity) will produce large errors of measurement. The Q angle represents the discrepancy between the pull of the quadriceps muscle and the anatomical position of the patellar tendon. The pull of the quadriceps is made up of the strong lateral pull of the vastus lateralis and a counteracting pull of the vastus medialis muscle. This vastus medialis oblique muscle therefore counteracts the tendency of the patella to sublux. Orthotics can affect the Q angle in the standing position; however, they have little effect on the Q angle in moving subjects.

51. Carpal tunnel syndrome:

a. False b. False c. True d. True e. False

Carpal tunnel syndrome (CTS) is an entrapment neuropathy of the median nerve at the wrist. It is seen in athletes who use their hands repetitively, and is often associated with a flexor tendonitis at the forearm or wrist. If an athlete develops a tendonitis distal to the flexor retinaculum, a trigger finger usually develops. If the flexor tendonitis occurs at the wrist the median nerve may become compromised with resulting carpal tunnel signs. The usual symptom is of tingling in the fingers, especially in the radial three and a half digits. The pain regularly wakes the subject at night, and the patient may describe shaking the finger to relieve the symptoms. Occasionally the pain travels up the arm, and it may travel as far as the shoulder in some cases. Tinnel's sign is not always positive, and some authors suggest that tapping on any nerve will in fact produce symptoms in normal individuals. Phalen's sign, which is forced volar flexion of the wrist for 90 seconds, usually reproduces the symptoms. The diagnosis is usually made by electrodiagnostic techniques, which usually show prolongation of the distal latency of the medial nerves' sensory and motor components. If the motor component is significantly compromised, then the abductor policis brevis muscle will also show evidence of denervation on needle EMG.

52. Lateral epicondylitis:

a. True b. False c. False d. False e. False

Lateral epicondylitis is a very common occupational and sports injury. The road to successful resolution of this injury involves relief of the painful symptoms of lateral elbow pain and rehabilitation of a usually weakened extensor forearm apparatus. Many modalities have been used to treat the painful extensor tendon and muscle mass prior to engaging in rehabilitation. Up to 85 per cent of steroid injections, up to 80 per cent of non-steroidal anti-inflammatory drugs, and 50 per cent of ultrasound treatments relieve the symptoms. Elbow straps should be worn in the acute phase of the injury and also following treatments such as steroid injection or physical modalities, as it will ensure adequate rest of the extensor mechanism following treatment. Following a steroid injection, the injected area should be treated as an acute musculo-tendon injury – with rest, ice and compression if necessary. Rehabilitation exercises or active sports activity should not be started for a minimum of 7–10 days, as the steroid injection may have a catabolic effect over this period of time and thus increase the likelihood of a local tissue rupture.

Further reading: Wiesner, S. L. (1991). Rehabilitation of elbow injuries in sports in physical medicine and rehabilitation clinics of North America. *Sports Med.*, **5**(1), 81–113.

53. Chronic low back pain:

a. False b. True c. True d. False e. False

Chronic low back pain is common among both the athletic and non-athletic populations, affecting up to 80 per cent of the population at some stage during their life. The causes are multifactorial. Athletes are potentially more at risk of low back pain due to the stresses their spine is placed under (repetitive loading, repetitive contact and sudden violent muscle contraction). Avoidance of low back pain syndromes can be achieved by establishing a correct trunk muscle function which in turn helps to protect the spine from injury. Normative data would suggest that extensor back muscles produce strength of between 90 per cent and 100 per cent of the body weight. This can be calculated by use of an isokinetic dynamometer, and is calculated in torque (foot pounds). Research would suggest that certain athletic groups such as rugby and football players, and the athletic population in general, produce larger torque values than non-athletes. Back muscle weakness is considered to be extensor muscle function below 64 per cent of the body weight. Levels below this are considered to be significantly weak, and are associated with chronic low back pain syndromes. Abnormal flexor to extensor ratios also signify chronic low back pain weakness. In a normal healthy back, the extensor muscles usually produce 30 per cent greater torque levels than the flexor or abdominal muscles. The trunk muscles can be restored to a normal level of function by a combination of co-ordination and endurance training. Various programmes, such as Mayer's Rehabilitation Program, incorporate both these strategies to restore a back to a normal level of function.

54. Achilles tendon injuries:

a. True b. False c. True d. False e. False

Achilles tendon injuries are commonly seen in athletes. Three quarters of Achilles tendon injuries affect the paratendon. The Achilles tendon consists of 30 per cent elastin, 48 per cent collagen and 21 per cent water. It is surrounded by a thin sheet called the epitenon; this is in turn surrounded by a second fine sheet called the peritenon. A potential space therefore exists between these two sheets, and inflammation that occurs at this site is referred to as a paratendinitis. Causes of Achilles tendon injury include direct trauma, training error, incorrect equipment (such as incorrectly fitting heel tabs) and anatomical factors (such as excessive ankle dorsiflexion, rear foot valgus in a flexible foot and rear foot varus in a rigid foot. The tendon itself adapts well to the stress of exercise. There is a normal ratio of the gastrocnemius complex to the Achilles tendon. As the gastrocnemius is hypertrophic, it is accompanied by an appropriate increase in the size and weight of the tendon, ensuring that the muscle to tendon ratio is maintained.

55. Legg–Calve–Perthes disease:

a. False b. False c. True d. True e. True

Legg–Calve–Perthes disease is a non-inflammatory disorder of the hip, which is thought to be due to disruption of the vascular supply to the femoral head. Legg–Calve–Perthes disease usually presents between the ages of 2 and 12 years, with the majority of cases occurring between 4 and 8 years of age. The incidence is higher in boys than girls. The condition usually presents as a painless limp after activity. The limp may worsen, and the patient may complain of pain in his hip, leg, groin or knee.

Legg–Calve–Perthes disease can be classified into four stages based on radiographic findings of the percentage involvement of the epiphysis. Plain radiographs can identify avascular necrosis. MRI and bone scanning may also allow an earlier diagnosis of ischaemic necrosis.

Treatment protocols involve regaining the full range of hip motion, and containment of the femoral head in the acetabulum via avarus osteotomy of the femur or an innominate osteotomy of the pelvis.

Further reading: Legg, A. T. (1910). An obscure affliction of the hip joint. *Boston Med. Surg. J.*, **162**, 202.

56. The rotator cuff syndrome:

a. False b. True c. True d. False e. True

The rotator cuff syndrome is a commonly encountered sporting injury. It usually involves a local tendon injury to one of the rotator cuff muscles with secondary impingement and, occasionally, a subacromial bursa. The most commonly injured tendon is the supraspinatus. Clinical examination is the key to a successful diagnosis. There is usually limitation in shoulder abduction and internal rotation with blocking, usually at a level of 90–100° of abduction. Resisted abduction frequently causes local anterior shoulder pain at the supraspinatus tendon insertion into the humeral head. The Hawkin's sign is helpful in identifying a supraspinatus impingement syndrome; the patient's forearm is internally rotated while it is forward flexed to 90°, and pain indicates a positive test. The Near's test is also used for identifying a rotator cuff impingement syndrome; the patient's shoulder is fully flexed to 180°, and the test is positive if there is pain at the end range of the arc. Stoddard's test is usually positive in cases of lateral epicondylitis; this involves resisted wrist extension, and a positive test exacerbates pain at the lateral epicondyle at the lateral extensor muscle mass of the forearm. Spurling's test is a clinical test to detect cervical nerve root involvement in cervical spine disease; the examiner applies rotational and compression forces downwards on the skull while rotating the head, and the test is positive if it recreates radicular pain.

57. Patellofemoral syndrome:

a. False b. False c. False d. False e. True

The patellofemoral syndrome is a very common and often confusing syndrome, and refers to anterior knee pain at the patellofemoral joint. The term chondromalacia patellae was frequently interchangeable with the patello-femoral syndrome; however, it is now established that chondromalacia patellae refers only to a degenerative change in the cartilage at the patellofemoral joint. There are two types of articular cartilage lesion at the patella: surface degeneration, which is commonly seen with age-related arthritis, and a second type affecting the deeper layers, characterized by basal degeneration.

Abnormally shaped or positioned patellae are associated with patello-femoral syndrome. Abnormalities of the ratio of the long axis and articular surface also increase the likelihood of patellofemoral syndrome. The patella itself increases the overall effectiveness of the extensor movement of the knee joint by approximately 50 per cent; however, in so doing it significantly increases the retropatellar compression force, and it is thought that this increased force may be a contributing factor to patellofemoral syndrome. The patellofemoral joint force will vary with activity: it is 0.5 times the body weight during walking, 2.5 times the body weight when stair ascending, 3.5 times the body weight when stair descending, and approximately half this level when rising from a squatting position.

Further reading: Fulkerson, J. P. (1997). *Disorders of the Patellofemoral Joint*. Lippincott Williams & Wilkins.

58. Heel spurs:

a. True b. True c. True d. False e. True

Heel spurs usually project from the medial tubercle of the calcaneous. The incidence of these spurs in asymptomatic individuals is between 10 and 30 per cent, and up to 75 per cent of individuals with painful heels also have heel spurs; however, 63 per cent of these individuals also have a spur on the non-painful side. The formation of the calcaneal spur is a result of the mechanical stress acting through the plantar fascia onto its origin at the calcaneum. Heel spurs are also observed with the seronegative arthropathies and rheumatoid arthritis, and in these cases the spurs are usually large and fluffy rather than the usually small traction spurs. There is a great deal of debate regarding the role of heel spurs in the production of pain; however, it is accepted that very large heel spurs may of themselves generate symptoms. Increased running distance and ankle plantar flexion are both associated factors in the development of heel spurs and heel pain.

Further reading: Taunton, J. E., Clement, D. B. and McNicol, K. (1982). Plantar fasciitis in runners. *Can. J. Appl. Sports Sci.*, **7**(1), 41-4.

59. Morton's metatarsalgia:

a. False b. True c. True d. False e. True

The syndrome of Morton's metatarsalgia results from damage to the interdigital nerve, usually between the third and fourth metatarsals, and was first described by Thomas G. Morton in 1876. It is an entrapment neuropathy, characterized by deposition of fibres rather than neural tissue followed by degeneration of the nerve fibre. The swelling is usually on the plantar surface of the intermetatarsal ligament. The patient usually presents with pain in the forefoot radiating into one or a number of toes, and paraesthesiae and numbness in adjacent toes. Symptoms are worsened by standing and walking, particularly when wearing shoes, and are characteristically relieved by sitting and removing the shoes. Women are more affected than men. Examination of the foot usually shows no foot deformities, and symptoms may be reproduced by palpation between the heads of the metatarsals or dorsiflexion of the metatarso-phalangeal joint. There may be a clinical sensory loss in the distribution of the plantar digital nerves. Two theories exist as to the pathogenesis of this condition: Morton's original description was that the interdigital nerves were pinched between the heads of adjacent metatarsals, and there is also a possibility that the nerve is traumatized when it is pressed and stretched between the firm anterior edge of the deep and the transverse metatarsal ligaments. Treatment involves a change of footwear; usually, flatter shoes are required. Metatarsal bars are also helpful, and pain relief can be achieved with corticosteroid and anaesthetic injections and carbamazepine. Excision of the plantar digital nerves and incising the deep intermetatarsal ligament are surgical options that are also occasionally required; however, surgery has the disadvantage of permanent loss of sensation around the affected toe. Occasionally, there is regrowth of a stump neuroma.

Further reading: Oh, S. J., Kim, H. S. and Ahmad, B. K. (1984). Electrophysiological diagnosis of interdigital neuropathy of the foot. *Musc. Nerve*, **7**(3), 218–25.

60. Iliopsoas injury:

a. False b. False c. False d. False e. False

Iliopsoas muscle injury is a source of groin pain among soccer players, the most common cause being that of an adductor tendonitis. It is caused by overuse inflammation rather than direct trauma. The pattern of pain is different from other causes of groin pain in that the pain is usually located in the lower abdominal quadrant lateral to the rectus abdominis muscle and above the inguinal ligament, and may radiate into the groin. The pain is aggravated by forced hip flexion against resistance. Treatment involves non-steroidal anti-inflammatories, rest, and iliopsoas flexibility and strengthening exercises. Occasionally, local steroid therapy is required via injection or iontophoresis.

Further reading: Mozes, M., Papa, M. Z. and Zweig, A. (1985). Iliopsoas injury in soccer players. *Br. J. Sports Med.*, **19**, 168–70.

61. Fractures associated with inversional injuries of the ankle joint:

a. True b. False c. True d. True e. True

Inversional ankle injuries are a common cause of morbidity in exercising individuals. Upwards of 59 per cent of individuals have problems associated with a single inversional injury 10 years following the initial trauma. One of the causes of an unresolved inversional ankle pathology is that of failure to diagnose an associated fracture. The ankle joint is made up of a mortise formed by the talus, the medial and lateral malleoli and the distal tibia. This ring of bone is vulnerable following an inversional or rotational ankle injury. In the cases of significant external rotation injuries of the ankle joint, excess stress is placed on the proximal fibula shaft, which may result in a local fibula fracture. This fracture can often be overlooked, as the main symptoms are around the ankle joint. A fractured proximal fibula in association with subluxation of the ankle joint and fracture of the medial malleolus or posterior malleolus, accompanied by disruption of the ankle mortise, is referred to as a Maissoneuve fracture. A twisted ankle can also result in fracture of the base of the 5th metatarsal. This fracture is usually transverse to the long axis of the metatarsal rather than longitudinal, which is usually associated with an unfused apophysis. The calcaneum bone can also be fractured in cases of significant inversional or rotational ankle injuries. An osteochondral fracture of the dome of the talus is a rare but frequently missed consequence of a plantar flexion inversional injury. The dome is wedged beneath the tibia and a shearing force is applied to its upper surface, which can result in an osteochondral injury. Clinically, there is pain on palpation over the dome of the talus, and specific talar views are required with, occasionally, bone scanning to identify an osteochondral defect.

62. Salter–Harris fractures:

a. True b. False c. True d. False e. True

The Salter–Harris fracture classification relates to fractures involving the growth plates of the unfused skeleton. Fractures are classified from 1 to 5 depending on their clinical importance; Salter–Harris type 1 injuries have a good prognosis, while type 5 have a poor prognosis. Type 1 fractures are across the growth plates with only very slight displacement of the epiphysis from the metaphysis; it is therefore often impossible to detect the pathology on plain X-rays. Type 2 fractures are through the metaphysis extending into the epiphyseal plate. Type 3 involves a fracture through the distal tibial epiphysis, extending into the epiphyseal plate; radiographs will often identify widening of the growth plate. Type 4 injuries involve the epiphyseal plate, the epiphysis and the metaphysis. Type 5 Salter–Harris injuries are impaction fractures of the entire growth plate; there is usually very little malalignment, and they can therefore be very difficult to diagnose from plain X-rays. The diagnosis is usually made from clinical suspicion and examination of the damaged bone. It is important not to miss a type 5 Salter–Harris fracture, as these injuries can result in premature diffusion of the growth plate with consequent limb shortening – this can occasionally also happen in type 4 injuries. Injuries to growth plates can cause significant morbidity to the young athlete. The risk of growth plate injuries is one of the causes of major concern for the young athlete who engages in unsupervised weight-lifting programmes; an accident while engaging in this type of activity can result in significant growth plate pathologies with subsequent disability and deformity due to unequal growth as a consequence of premature fusion of growth plates.

63. Avulsion fractures:

a. False b. False c. True d. False e. False

An avulsion fracture is caused when a bony fragment or apophysis is pulled away from the parent bone. It can occur at the site of the insertion of a tendon or ligament, and is frequently observed in the sporting community as a result of excessive muscle contraction or an abnormal degree of movement at a joint. It may also be caused by repetitive strain or overuse. This is the case with an ischial tuberosity avulsion fracture, which is commonly seen in midfield field players who are constantly twisting and turning. This results in excessive force of the adductor magnus muscle on the ischial tuberosity, with resulting avulsion. Avulsion fractures can also occur around the hip. Avulsion at the anterior superior iliac spine is usually caused by repetitive or excessive pull by the sartorius muscle. The anterior inferior iliac spine avulsion fracture is caused by the excessive or repetitive pull of the rectus femorous muscle. The medial epicondyle can also be a rare site for avulsion fracture. This is caused by the excessive pull of the forearm flexor muscles, which are inserted at the medial epicondyle. If the medial epicondyle becomes displaced, it may lie within the elbow joint and be misinterpreted as being a normal ossification centre in the younger athlete. A rule of thumb worth remembering when examining the younger athlete with a suspected medial epicondyle avulsion is to visualize the trochlear ossification centre. The trochlea ossifies after the medial epicondyle; therefore, if the trochlea is observed on X-ray, there must also be an ossified medial epicondyle visible.

64. Bennett's fracture:

a. True b. False c. False d. False e. False

A Bennett's fracture occurs at the base of the thumb, and can cause articular damage at this site. It is usually caused by a forceful hyperextension injury to the thumb, which results in a local avulsion fracture of the metacarpus and disruption of the CMC joint at the base of the thumb. This fracture, along with other metacarpal fractures, is frequently seen in athletes who engage in falling sports and is common in skiers, bicycle riders and gymnasts. Radiological findings reveal a fracture at the base of the first metacarpal extending into the joint surface, with accompanying dislocation of the carpo-metacarpal joint. The metacarpal is pulled dorsally and radially by the pull of the abductor policis longus muscle. Treatment involves careful assessment of the fracture. If dislocation also occurs, open reduction and internal fixation is required and the thumb is then immobilized in a cast for 4–6 weeks. The athlete is usually ready to return to contact sport 8–10 weeks after the injury.

Further reading: McCue, F. C., Baugher, W. H. and Kunland, D. N. (1979). Hand and wrist injuries in the athlete. *Am. J. Sport. Med.*, (**7**), 275.

65. Ulnar collateral ligament injuries of the elbow:

a. False b. True c. True d. True e. True

Ulnar collateral ligament injuries are commonly seen in athletes who participate in throwing and racket sports. An ulnar collateral ligament injury is usually caused by repetitive valgus stress on the elbow, which increases the tension on the ulnar collateral ligament. Injury or weakness of the elbow flexors and pronator muscles increase the stresses that are transferred to the ligament. Throwing sports often involve rapid elbow extension with valgus stress and rotation, resulting in medial traction and lateral compression on the ligament, and injury. Occasionally the repetitive loading on the ligament can result in an osseous formation, which can cause an ulnar neuropathy on the elbow. The initial treatment is conservative, with rest, non-steroidal anti-inflammatories and strengthening of the flexor pronator muscle complex. Throwing and racket technique may also be altered or augmented. If the ligament has been completely ruptured or there is a poor response to conservative therapy, surgery may be contemplated; this usually involves an autograft using the palmaris longus or plantaris tendon.

Further reading: Fox, G. M., Jebson, P. J. L. and Orwin, J. F. (1995). Overuse injuries of the elbow. *Phys. Sports Med.*, **23**(8).

66. Spondylolysis:

a. False b. False c. False d. False e. True

Spondylolysis affects approximately 5 per cent of the North American population, and is usually caused by a stress fracture of the pars interarticularis. It can, however, also occur as an acute fracture, and may be a site of a lytic lesion in an older subject. The L5 level is the most commonly affected; however, the L4 and, to a lesser extent, L3 levels can also be involved. Less than half the patients with spondylolysis will develop spondylolisthesis, which is a forward slip of the upper vertebrae on the lower vertebrae. Oblique radiographs usually demonstrate the break in the pars interarticularis referred to as the Scottie dog defect, although lateral X-rays will pick up about 85 per cent of the spondylolysis. If plain radiographs fail to pick up the lesion, then bone scanning or spectscanning usually show increased activity in the region of the pars interarticularis. The majority of spondylolyses are chronic when first detected, and treatment is therefore usually supervised rest and activity modification. If symptoms persist after 2 months, cast immobilization for 2–3 months is often recommended. Sports activity is restricted during this period. Surgery is occasionally indicated for spondylolysis if symptoms persist despite a 12-week period of cast immobilization, if there is spondylolisthesis of more than 50 per cent displacement and if the symptons are recurrent.

Further reading: Steiner, M. E. and Micheli, L. J. (1985). Treatment of symptomatic spondylolysis and spondylolisthesis with the modified Boston brace. *Spine*, **10**(10), 937–43.

67. Acromioclavicular injuries:

a. False b. True c. True d. True e. True

Acromioclavicular joint injuries commonly occur among the athletic community, and the majority are caused by landing on the point of the shoulder. However, injuries can also be caused by a blow from behind when the ipsilateral arm is fixed on the ground, which results in the clavicle being driven forward from the acromion. A fall on the outstretched hand can also cause injury at the acromioclavicular joint, due to the backwards and upward force on the acromion. The acromioclavicular joint is the second most commonly dislocated area around the shoulder; the gleno-humeral is the most common and the sternoclavicular joint the least. Acromioclavicular joint injuries are based on the extent of the ligament injury. Rockwood and Young have produced a grading system that refers to the levels as types rather than grades. Type 1 is a sprain involving a partial disruption of the acromioclavicular ligament and capsule. There is usually point tenderness over the joint, and laxity of the joint is absent. Type 2 consists of a rupture of the acromioclavicular ligaments and capsule, with an incomplete injury to the coracoclavicular ligament. There is usually minimal acromioclavicular joint subluxation. Type 3 exhibits complete tearing of the acromioclavicular and coracoclavicular ligaments. The acromioclavicular joint is usually dislocated, and deformity is also obvious with the distal end of the clavicle easy to palpate. Type 4 dislocations consist of a displaced clavicle penetrating posteriorly into the trapezius muscle. An Alexander view X-ray (scapular lateral view) will reveal the posterior displacement of the clavicle. Clinically, the condition can be observed by viewing the patient from above the shoulder joint. Type 5 dislocations are similar to type 3, but with a greater coracoclavicular interval (usually 100 per cent greater than the uninjured side). Type 6 injuries are rare, but result in the patient's clavicle being displaced inferiorly to the coracoid process.

Further reading: Rockwood, C. A. and Young, D. C. (1990). Disorders of the acromioclavicular joint. In *The Shoulder* (C. A. Rockwood and F. A. Matsen, eds), pp. 413–76. W. B. Saunders.

68. Patellofemoral pain:

a. True b. True c. False d. False e. True

The patellofemoral syndrome is a descriptive term that is now regularly used to describe anterior knee pain of any aetiology, but more frequently those syndromes without any significant gross anatomical changes in the articular cartilage of the patella. Malalignment accounts for the majority of cases of patellofemoral syndrome; however, trauma (such as patellar fractures, patellar dislocations and tendon ruptures) can also be included under the umbrella of patellofemoral syndrome. Late effects of trauma such as osteoarthritis are also included in this group, as are medial schelf plica disorder, tendonopathies, peri-patellar bursitis and osteochondritis dissecans. Patellofemoral syndrome often has a typical presentation; a young adult who has anterior knee pain. The pain is usually dull, with episodes of sharp pain exacerbated by going up and down stairs. The patient does not necessarily have to have a history of sports participation, and may give a history of the 'theatre-goer's' sign – i.e. anterior knee pain after prolonged sitting. Recent data has suggested that patients with a history of Osgood–Schlatter's disease have an elevated risk of developing patellofemoral syndrome. Eighty-two per cent of conservative treatment is reported as being successful in the treatment of patellofemoral syndrome, and only after exhaustive use of medical treatments should surgery be considered. Surgical options are often mainly geared towards local treatment of inflammatory tissue at the patellofemoral joint, or realignment procedures such as lateral release of the retinaculum or tibial tubercle transfer.

Further reading: Galea, A. M. and Albers, J. M. (1994). Patellofemoral pain. *Phys. Sports Med.*, **22**(4).

69. Malalignments associated with the patellofemoral syndrome:

a. True b. False c. True d. True e. True

The majority of cases of patellofemoral syndrome are due to malalignments. The most common malalignment disorder is a weakened vastus medialis oblique muscle; however, an altered Q angle, in particular elevated Q angles (in both males and females), increases the likelihood of maltracking of the patellofemoral joint. Other anatomical malalignments affecting the lower limb have also being implicated in patellofemoral syndrome, including pes planus or pes cavus, and tightness of the lateral retinaculum, ilio-tibial band or hamstring. Congenital malalignments are also important to identify. Patella beja and patella alta have been implicated in patellofemoral syndrome and, more recently, three patella morphological types have been identified. The cyrano-shaped patella has been noted to have a particular increased incidence of patellofemoral syndrome.

Further reading: Insall, J. (1979). Chondromalacia patellae, patella malalignment syndrome. *Orthop. Clin. N. America*, **10**(1), 117–27.

70. Levator scapula syndrome:

a. False b. False c. True d. True e. True

The levator scapula muscle takes its origin from the transverse processes of the cervical vertebrae C1–C4. It has a broad insertion into the supero-medial border of the scapula, and receives its nerve supply from the 3rd and 4th cervical nerve root and its blood supply from the transverse and descending cervical arteries. The levator scapula syndrome presents as a generalized periscapular pain. It may be associated with direct trauma, and is regularly related to lifting occupations. The condition can be aggravated by sailing, golfing, weight-lifting and combat sports, and is also often seen following a flexion–extension decelerating automobile accident. The levator scapula is a deep structure, and therefore palpation requires patients to be placed in a prone position, supporting their body weight on abducted elbows approximately shoulder width apart. This exposes the scapulae, and the superomedial border can then be examined. Levator scapula syndrome can mimic many conditions, such as gall bladder disease, pancreatitis and lung cancer, as well as cervical radiculopathy and cervical spondylosis. Treatment of this painful condition consists of stretching the injured structure. The ice and stretch modality is often most beneficial, using either crushed ice in a polythene bag or ethyl chloride prior to stretching. Other physical modalities can also give pain relief. Occasionally steroid injection is warranted in the more painful cases, and the injection position for the patient is similar to that used for examination. Great care must be taken in performing this injection, as the danger of pneumothorax is considerable.

Further reading: Estwanik, J. J. (1989). Levator scapulae syndrome. *Phys. Sports Med.*, **17**(10), 57.

71. Popliteal tendonitis:

a. False b. True c. True d. True e. True

The popliteus muscle has three origins:

1. The lateral femoral condyle
2. The fibres from the fibular head, and
3. Oblique fibres from the lateral meniscus, posterior cruciate, posterior capsule and ligaments of Winslow.

The fibres form a thick muscle belly, which inserts in the postero-superior part of the tibial condyle. The muscle acts in combination with the posterior cruciate ligament to prevent anterior displacement of the femur. The muscle also allows retraction of the posterior horn of the lateral meniscus during knee flexion, and acts as an internal rotator of the tibia. The popliteal tendon is usually injured by overuse, and downhill running and over-striding put particular stress on this muscle. The athlete may present with posterior knee pain that occurs during activity. There may be specific pain during knee flexion, and walking with a straight leg can eliminate some of the posterior knee pain. Treatment involves activity modification and symptom reduction with non-steroidal anti-inflammatories and physical therapy. This condition is frequently confused with a Baker's cyst or a posterior horn injury of the meniscus. Careful examination of the popliteus muscle is best achieved by relaxing the hamstrings by placing the patient's leg over the examiner's shoulder, allowing easier access to the popliteus muscle and tendon.

Further reading: Basmajian, J. V. and Lovejoy, J. F. (1971). Functions of the popliteus muscle in man. *J. Bone Joint Surg.*, **53**, 557-62.

Special groups

72. The young athlete:

a. False b. True c. True d. True e. False

Treating child and adolescent athletes requires a healthy suspicion of underlying bony injury. Children's ligaments are generally stronger than their growth plates and surrounding bones; therefore, significant injuries to knees and ankles frequently result in bony or growth plate injuries rather than the ligamentous pattern usually observed in an adult. In the case of the knee, a hyper-extension twisting injury may result in an avulsion fracture at the tibial eminence rather than an anterior cruciate ligament substance tear, which is likely in an adult. Apophysitis injuries are also common among young athletes. An apophysitis is a site of the growth cartilage where the musculo-tendinous unit attaches to the bone. Apophysitis can occur due to direct trauma such as a forceful muscle contraction, which can cause an avulsion fracture, or micro-trauma, which results in irritation and inflammation of the apophysitis. Sever's disease is a calcaneal apophysitis, which is a common complaint in the athletic child and adolescent. It is usually seen at the age of 12 years in boys and 11 years in girls; the typical picture is that of a young boy complaining of heel pain exacerbated by activity. Clinical examination may reveal tenderness on lateral and medial compression of the calcaneus. This is usually a self-limiting condition, which occasionally needs cast immobilization. Iselin's disease is a very rare traction apophysitis at the base of the 5th metatarsal, and usually presents with pain on the lateral side of the foot when running or jumping. Radiology may show an enlarged apophysis with abnormal ossification. Treatment involves rest and strengthening of the inverter and dorsiflexor muscle groups, and stretching of the evertor and plantiflexor muscle groups.

Further reading: Micheli, L. J. and Fehlandt, A. F. Jnr. (1992). Overuse injuries to tendons and apophyses in children and adolescents. *Clin. Sports Med.*, **11**(4), 713–26.

73. Exercise and ageing:

a. True b. False c. True d. False e. True

Many athletes continue to exercise into their middle and late years. Physiological function, however, alters as we get older. As we age, the peak performance in both endurance and strength activities decreases by about 1–2 per cent per year, starting in the late twenties. The VO_2 max decreases by approximately 10 per cent per decade, starting in the late teens for women and the mid-twenties for men. This is mainly due to a decrease in cardiorespiratory function. Maximum heart rate, stroke volume and cardiac output all decrease with age. It is thought to be due to both inactivity and physical ageing. The respiratory vital capacity and forced expiratory volume decrease linearly with age; the residual volume increases, and the total lung capacity remains unchanged. These pulmonary changes that are associated with advancing years are primarily caused by a loss of elasticity in the lungs and chest wall.

Further reading: Pollock, M. L., Foster, C. and Rod, J. L. (1987). Effect of age and training on aerobic capacity and body composition of master athletes. *J. Appl. Physiol.*, **62**(2), 725–31.

74. Osteochondritis dissecans:

a. True b. False c. False d. False e. False

Osteochondritis dissecans of the knee is caused by a necrotic area of subchondral bone, which often results in separation of a fragment of cartilage and subchondral bone from an articular surface. It most commonly affects the medial femoral condyle; however, the lateral femoral condyle and patella can also be affected. Patients usually present during their adolescent or early adult years, and often give a history of knee pain and swelling exacerbated by activity. The diagnosis can be confirmed by radiological findings. These should include antero-posterior (AP), lateral and axial views. The tunnel view is particularly useful in visualizing lesions that may not be seen by the standard radiographs. MRI is also helpful in determining the size of the lesion.

The cause of osteochondritis dissecans is unknown, although a traumatic cause has been proposed. It is suggested that the medial femoral condyle may be injured by repetitive trauma from the medial tibial spine, and that repetitive stresses during activity from traction on the posterior ligament may be a cause of this injury in the athletic population. The prognosis is better for younger patients and individuals with smaller lesions.

Further reading: Wilson, J. N. (1967). A diagnostic sign in osteochondritis dissecans of the knee. *J. Bone Joint Surg.*, **49**(3), 477–80.

75. Exercise and diabetes:

a. True b. False c. True d. False e. False

The benefits of exercise for patients with diabetes have been known for hundreds of years. Research has indicated that improved glucose transport occurs after physical exercise. Regular physical activity may lower resting heart rate and blood pressure as well as helping to maintain lean body mass, an aid in weight reduction. In addition to the physiological benefits, research has also indicated that diabetics who regularly exercise will improve their self-esteem and self-confidence. There has been some variation in the effects of exercise on diabetics' lipid profiles, and there is only possibly a beneficial effect on the lipid profiles. There has also been variation in the research findings concerning haemoglobin A1. Some studies indicate an exercise-related decrease in both haemoglobin A1 and blood glucose; however, this has not been proven in all studies and can therefore only be considered a possible beneficial effect.

76. Absolute contraindications for exercise during pregnancy:

a. True b. True c. False d. False e. False

Exercise during pregnancy is now recommended by most obstetricians. Contraindications for exercise during pregnancy have been established by the American College of Obstetrics and Gynecology. These include absolute contraindications (such as heart disease, ruptured membranes, placenta praevia, incompetent cervix and a history of three or more spontaneous abortions) and relative contraindications (including high blood pressure, anaemia, thyroid disease and diabetes, palpitations, a history of bleeding during pregnancy and an extremely sedentary life style).

Further reading: American College of Obstetricians and Gynecologists (1985). *Exercise During Pregnancy and the Postnatal Period. Home Exercise Program.* ACOG.

77. Female incontinence and exercise:

a. False b. True c. True d. False e. False

Incontinence affects people of all ages, and women are twice as likely as men to be incontinent. A survey assessing the prevalence of exercise incontinence suggested that 47 per cent of regularly exercising women report some degree of incontinence, and this correlated positively with the number of vaginal deliveries. Over 20 per cent of those noting incontinence were nulliparous. Higher impact exercises, such as running and aerobics, resulted in a greater incidence of incontinence, with an incidence of more than 35 per cent reported. Lower impact activities, such as swimming and racket ball, reported levels of just over 10 per cent, and weight-lifting had the smallest incidence, with only 7 per cent reporting incontinence. Further research has indicated that specific sports have very high levels of incontinence; these include gymnastics and basketball. The key to treating this frequently undiagnosed problem is that of exercise modification, including planning exercise routes with access to lavatory facilities and limiting fluid intake. Exercise aimed at improving the neuromuscular function of the pelvic floor muscle complex has also been shown to be helpful. Occasionally, surgical or pharmacological treatments are required.

Further reading: Nygaard, I., Delancey, J. O. and Arnsdorf, L. (1990). Exercise and incontinence. *Obst. Gynecol.*, **75**(5), 848–51.

78. Restrictive eating behaviour:

a. False b. False c. False d. True e. False

Restrictive eating disorder is common among active and athletic women. Restrictive eating behaviour can range from poor nutrition to voluntary starvation, and from a subclinical syndrome to frank anorexia nervosa. Obsessional and compulsive behaviour are observed both in the patient's eating pattern and in normal daily activities. Athletes who restrict food intake often do not meet the criteria for diagnosis of anorexia nervosa. The physical symptoms that are commonly encountered include dry skin, brittle hair and nails, cold intolerance, amenorrhoea, constipation, and a sensation of bloating after eating. The physical signs include discoloration of hands and feet, low blood pressure, laguno hair, bradycardia, hypothermia and decreased subcutaneous fat.

Further reading: Vigersky, R. A., Anderson, A. E. and Thompson, R. H. (1977). Hypothalamic dysfunction in secondary amenorrhea associated with simple weight loss. *N. Engl. J. Med.*, **297**(21), 1141–5.

79. Restrictive eating behaviour:

a. False b. False c. False d. True e. True

The common laboratory findings associated with restrictive eating disorder, which is an eating disorder frequently observed in active and athletic women, include normal FSH levels, low/normal LH levels and normal T4 and TSH levels, although T3 is often low due to decreased peripheral conversion of T4 to T3. This is thought to be due to reduced calorie intake. The blood urea is often elevated. Urinalysis can provide evidence of proteinuria and haematuria. A blood picture can show leucopenia, anaemia and thrombocytopenia. Individuals who fluid overload, which can be associated with restrictive eating disorder, may also show evidence of hyponatraemia.

Further reading: Pameroy, C. and Mitchell, J. E. (1992). Medical issues in the eating disorders. In *Eating, Body Weight and Performance in Athletes, Disorders of Modern Society* (K. D. Brownell, J. Rodan and J. H. Wilmore, eds). Lea and Febiger.

80. Pregnancy and exercise:

a. False b. True c. True d. False e. True

Up to 20 per cent of women considering pregnancy take regular exercise, and these women also plan to continue exercising during their pregnancy. The question regarding the safety and appropriateness of exercise during pregnancy remains unanswered, with the dilemma relating to any potential danger to the foetus. In pregnancy, the concern is that of exercise-induced hyperthermia, which may cause abortion or congenital abnormalities; however, the association between elevated maternal temperature and congenital malformations remains unproven. The blood vessels that supply the uterus are part of the splanchnic circulation. As training intensity increases, the splanchnic blood flow decreases and the uterine blood flow will therefore also decrease. The concern is that this reduced blood flow may impair nutrients and oxygen available to the foetus. There is also a concern that the fall in myometrial oxygen delivery may stimulate contractions, leading to pre-term labour. As body weight increases during pregnancy, it is suggested that stresses may increase on musculoskeletal structures. Despite this increased potential risk, there has been no particular increase in injury rates noted among females who take exercise during pregnancy. Pregnancy outcome data in individuals who take exercise is positive; despite this, the recommendations for exercise during pregnancy remain cautious and it is suggested that low intensity exercise with a heart rate below 140 or 150 be carried out for not more than 15–20 minutes. It is also recommended that the exerciser should avoid sudden, 'jerky' types of exercises.

Further reading: American College of Obstetricians and Gynecologists (1985). *Exercise During Pregnancy and the Postnatal Period.* ACOG.

81. Rugby union injuries:

a. False b. False c. True d. False e. True

Rugby union injuries are on the increase. A survey of rugby injuries in 1989 showed an incidence of one significant injury requiring medical attention per 31 player appearances, implying that there is approximately one significant injury per rugby match (30 players). In August 1995 rugby union football became a professional sport, and with it has come an increased injury rate. It is well established that professional sport has a significantly higher incidence of injury than recreational or amateur sport. Already, rugby union has a similar injury incidence and profile to that in American football and rugby league, with the knee, lower limb and shoulder being the most commonly affected injury sites. The playing position injury incidences have also changed. In the 1960s and 1970s, the back row players and scrum halves were the most frequently injured. In the present game, it is the centres and the full backs that are most frequently injured. This is due to the changes in the laws of rugby, which encourage defensive players to 'run the ball' out of defence in an offensive play. The change in kicking the ball directly into touch has also ensured a more fluid game, and a higher incidence of high-speed contact situations. With greater conditioning of players and larger, stronger players participating, it is likely that there will be further increases in the injury rates in this traditional field sport.

Further reading: O'Brien, C. P. (1992). Rugby injuries in the Leinster province of Ireland. *Br. J. Sports Med.*, **26**(4), 243-4.

82. Skateboarding:

a. False b. True c. True d. True e. False

Skateboarding is now one of the most popular recreational pursuits. It first became popular in the 1960s, when it was used as a means for surfers to practise their manoeuvres in colder weather. Over 50 per cent of skateboard injuries are fractures to the extremities, with the radius and ulna being the most commonly injured sites. Thirty per cent of skateboarding injuries occur on streets and highways and, although only 3 per cent of skateboard injuries involve motor vehicles, over half of all deaths related to skateboarding are associated with motor vehicle accidents. Prevention of injuries in this ever-increasing recreational pursuit involves advice regarding appropriate instruction for beginners prior to embarking on this hazardous pursuit. Care regarding equipment is also important in preventing injuries, and the board, bindings and skateboard trucks should all be checked regularly for wear and damage. The wearing of protective gear is particularly important in the novice skateboarder, and helmets, knee pads, elbow pads and gloves should all be worn in an effort to prevent the trauma of falling, which is part and parcel of this activity. There is also the important issue of the psychological make-up and culture of skateboarding to consider. This activity can be referred to as an extreme urban sport, and risk-taking is part and parcel of it. It was further popularized at the Centennial Olympic Games of 1996, where the closing ceremony demonstrated many of the death-defying activities of this new urban sport. Attempting any of these extreme manoeuvres without the appropriate skill will undoubtedly increase injury incidence. It is also important to understand the vocabulary of the skateboarding fraternity, in an effort to get over the message regarding safety. 'Goofy foot' refers to the natural tendency of a few people to ride a skateboard with the right foot forward rather than the left (which is the normal pattern), and an 'ollie' implies becoming airborne without a jump by lifting first the front foot and then the rear while springing off the tail of the board. Any physician who has an interest or deals with individuals who participate in this type of activity should be well-versed in the vocabulary in order to fully understand patients and be understood by them.

Further reading: Cass, D. T. and Ross, F. (1990). Skateboard injuries. *Med. J. Aust.*, **153**(3), 140, 143–4.

83. Head injuries in soccer:

a. False b. True c. True d. True e. True f. False

Head injuries account for 5–10 per cent of all soccer-related injuries, and fatal head injuries have been reported on rare occasions. Younger players are more susceptible to head injuries, and it is felt that this may be due to a poor heading technique among more inexperienced soccer players. The symptoms can include headache, irritability, dizziness, insomnia, impaired hearing and memory loss. The mechanisms of injury include improper heading of a football, head to head contact, and a ball travelling at high velocity striking a player's head. The majority of the injuries occur when the player is heading the ball, and it is thought that this may have a cumulative affect on an individual over a playing career. Research has indicated that professional soccer players head the ball five times on average per game, and this can add up to 5000 impacts in a 15-year career. Goalkeepers too can experience head injuries when they strike fellow players, the surface or the goal posts in the course of play.

Further reading: Fields, K. B. (1989). Head injuries in soccer. *Phys. Sports Med.*, **17**(1), 69–73.

84. Breaststroker's knee:

a. False b. True c. True d. True e. False

Breaststroker's knee is an overuse injury that selectively affects the medial collateral ligament of the knee, usually at the femoral attachment. It is caused by the forces applied in the sequence of the whip kick of this stroke, which follows a sequence of knee extension followed by valgus stress terminating with an external rotatory stress forced on this ligament. Unfortunately, to prevent the recurrence of this overuse injury, the kick may have to be modified so there is less external rotation of the tibia. Alternatively, the breaststroker may have to introduce other styles into their training programmes.

Further reading: Kennedy, J. C., Hawkins, R. and Krissoff, W. B. (1978). Orthopaedic manifestations of swimming. *Am. J. Sports Med.*, **6**, 309–22.

85. Snowboarding injuries:

a. True b. False c. False d. True e. False

Snowboarding is fast becoming one of the most popular winter sports. Snowboarders slalom down slopes while standing sideways on a board, and the position is similar to that of Hawaiian surfing. Snowboarding injury rates are similar to those in Alpine skiing, and up to 50 per cent of participants can be affected. Injuries are evenly distributed between the upper and lower limbs, with the wrist being the most commonly injured site. The wearing of special footwear affects the injury rates; 75 per cent of participants wear soft footwear with no hard shell, while the remaining 25 per cent wear footwear with a shell. Those individuals wearing hard shell boots are more likely to injure their knees, while those wearing soft boots are more likely to injure their ankles. The most common type of accident is a fall, with collisions being the least frequent type of accident. The actual mechanism of injury is usually that of a direct blow.

Further reading: Ganong, R. B. Heneveld, E. H., Beranek, S. R. et al. (1992). Snowboarding injuries. *Phys. Sports Med.*, **20**(12).

86. Physiological function and ageing:

a. True b. True c. False d. True e. False

Ageing is associated with a variety of metabolic and physiological changes. Reduced function in major organs and changes in cardiovascular and muscular performance have all been associated with advancing years. Maximum oxygen uptake declines at a rate of 1 per cent per year after the third decade of life, and isometric and dynamic muscle strength starts to decrease after the fifth decade. The decline in the exercise capacities observed with advancing years parallel the decline seen in the musculoskeletal and cardiorespiratory systems, and the decrease in cardiorespiratory function and reduced muscle mass and strength observed with advancing years mimic the decline noted in individuals who are bed bound. Therefore, the relevant importance of ageing per se versus the well-documented age-related decline in voluntary physical activity cannot be fully separated. Reduction in physiological performance may not be completely caused by the ageing process per se, but rather by a reduction in activity in the older age group. This older age group will make up a significant proportion of the population in the 21st century, and it is estimated that the geriatric age group (i.e. those over 65 years of age) will make upwards of 20 per cent of the North American population in the year 2030. The various physiological changes occur at different rates. There is a slowly progressive loss of lean tissue until the age of 65, followed by a more rapid decline. The aerobic function appears to reduce more rapidly following the third decade, and actual muscle function starts to decline in the fifth decade. With an increasing ageing population, it is therefore essential that this older population is encouraged to increase activity on an ongoing basis in order to try to help to reduce the decline in their exercise capacities.

Further reading: Aniansson, A. and Gustafssone, F.(1981). Physical training in elderly men. *Clin. Physiol.*, **1**, 87–98.

87. Frostbite:

a. True b. True c. True d. True e. False

Frostbite is a local destruction of superficial tissue, caused by freezing of extracellular water and dehydration damage to the exposed part. Frostbite usually occurs at 11 to 12°C. Contributory factors include over-tight garments and local vasoconstriction, which may occur in individuals who are cigarette smokers. Low air temperatures and exposure to high winds are also contributory factors. The initial treatment should be re-warming the affected area; however, following this the affected part should be kept cool to minimize the metabolic demand to the affected area. Untreated frostbite is commonly followed by gangrene.

Further reading: Shephard, R. J. (1988). Cold. In *The Olympic Book of Sports Medicine* (A. Dirix, H. G. Knuttgen and K. Tittel, eds). Blackwell Science.

88. Resistance training for the middle-aged adult:

a. True b. True c. False d. True e. True

Muscle strength and endurance are significant elements in an exercise programme for the middle-aged adult. These individuals are particularly in need of this type of conditioning, as they have increased leisure time and require adequate muscle function for lifting grandchildren, carrying luggage, pulling golf carts and working at DIY and gardening. Until recently, the majority of exercise programmes for individuals in the 50 to 65 year age group recommended aerobic type activity to the detriment of resistance training. Recent research has shown that, performed appropriately, resistance activity does not adversely affect either cardiovascular status or blood pressure. However, specific care must be taken with individuals with poor left ventricular function, and pure isometric contractions should be avoided as this may result in left ventricular decompensation. Isokinetic activity would appear to be an alternative, as the resistance alters automatically to the applied force and may therefore have a less significant effect on the left ventricular function. Dynamic low to moderate resistance exercise for large muscles is recommended. The most difficult element in prescribing resistance exercise is selecting an initial starting weight, and both 30 per cent and 80 per cent of a maximal lift have been recommended as possible starting levels. However, a more workable approach is to select the lightest weight on a free-standing resistance machine, and steadily work up to a level where 13–15 repetitions can be performed comfortably. Having achieved a level where 15 or more repetitions can be performed comfortably for three or four sets, the resistance can be increased. An adequate rest to work ratio should also be encouraged to avoid muscle fatigue, and an appropriate ratio would be 1 : 1 for those beginning resistance exercise. Free weights should be avoided until sufficient skill has been developed using weights machines. Free weights have the added advantage of improving muscle co-ordination as well as muscle strength and endurance; therefore, free weights are recommended for the more active exercisers who wish to improve their sports performance.

Further reading: O'Brien, C. P. (1997). The appropriate level of exercise for the middle-aged man and woman. *Modern Medicine of Ireland.*

Exercise prescription

89. Endurance exercise:

a. False b. True c. True d. False e. True

It is now well known that endurance exercise is associated with a beneficial effect on cardiovascular risk. In particular, cholesterol and lipid profiles can be improved by regular endurance activity, and levels of HDL-cholesterol, HDL2-cholesterol and apoprotein A1, which are all negatively associated with the development of coronary vascular disease, are increased by aerobic activity. LDL cholesterol, which is positively associated with the development of coronary vascular disease, may be either increased or decreased by aerobic activity. Exercise is also associated with variations in circulating hormones. Aldosterone is increased via the renin–angiotensin pathway, which is sensitive to aerobic exercise, and this increased aldosterone has the effect of increasing the intravascular circulating volume. As a result, athletes who regularly engage in aerobic activities may have evidence of physiological anaemia on their blood picture.

Further reading: Leaf, D. A., Bland, D. and Schaad, D. (1992). The relationship of total and leisure-time physical activity to coronary artery disease risk factors in medical students. *Med. Exer. Nutr. Health*, **1**(4), 208-216.

90. Proper bicycle fit:

a. True b. False c. True d. True e. False

Cycling is now one of the most popular recreational pursuits. The proper set up of the bike is intended to reduce biomechanical stresses on the lower body, and to maximize performance. Inappropriate bicycle set up can increase the incidence of musculoskeletal disease, and up to 10 per cent of competitive cyclists experience low back discomfort with another 10 per cent experiencing neck discomfort.

There are some simple measurements that should always be made to ensure the proper bicycle fit. The frame size should be such that there is a 2.5–5 cm clearance between the rider's crotch and the top of the tube of the bicycle. The saddle height should be such as to allow slight knee flexion of 10–15° with the pedal in the 6 o'clock position. The seat position is determined by placing the pedals in the 3 o'clock and 9 o'clock positions, with the balls of the feet centred on the pedal spindle. From this position, a plumb line is drawn from the anterior patella of the forward knee and this should bisect the pedal spindle. The handlebar height should be at a level with or just below the top of the seat. The handlebar reach is the distance from the front tip of the saddle to the horizontal portion of the handlebars, and the correct reach is determined by placing the elbow against the front seat and extending the arm towards the handlebars. The extended fingers should just touch the handlebars.

Further reading: Mellon, M. B. (1988). *Office Management of Sports Injuries and Athletic Problems.* Hanley and Belfus Inc.

91. Normal hormonal responses to exercise:

a. True b. False c. True d. True e. False

During prolonged exercise, there is a steady decline in plasma glucose and a decline in the release of insulin. This is associated with a progressive increase in glucagon; this hormone increases hepatic glycogenolysis, which in turn increases plasma glucose for the exercising muscles. There is also an increase in catecholamines, which is dependent on the intensity of the exercise. The increased catecholamines reduce insulin secretion, increase muscle glycogen breakdown and enhance hepatic glycoglucolysis. The increased catecholamines play a role in increasing tissue lipolysis. Cortisol and growth hormone are also increased during exercise; they potentiate the catecholamine effect and also impair the cellular action of insulin.

Further reading: Galbo, H., Holst, J. J. and Christensen, N. J. (1975). Glucagon and plasma catecholamine response to graded and prolonged exercise in man. *J. Appl. Physiol.*, **38**(1), 70-76.

92. Exercise for weight loss:

a. False b. True c. False d. True e. False

Obesity can be defined as a body fat percentage of greater than 25 per cent in males. It is an increasing problem among the western population, despite a significant reduction in calorie intake over the past three decades to below 3,000 calories per day. The key to successful exercising in the overweight population is high frequency, longer duration activity at a lower intensity. In short, high volume exercise programmes have the most beneficial effect.

Motivating the overweight individual to exercise is an important element in achieving a weight loss and health gain. Overweight athletes may be self-conscious regarding their poor athletic performance and have general feelings of lack of self-esteem; advising them to participate in group activities may therefore improve compliance. The actual mode of activity should be one that has a low skill level. Sports such as tennis have high skill levels, and overweight exercisers may have insufficient aptitude to gain a reasonable exercise benefit. Overweight exercisers also have the added problems of injury, discomfort and pain associated with activity due to their larger body weight, and activities such as stationary cycling, swimming, water aerobics and rowing should be selected, as these will reduce the stresses on joints and soft tissues. Subjects should be encouraged to start on a walking programme and, over a period of weeks, build this up to 60 minutes a day at a moderate intensity (i.e. at a level where a conversation can comfortably be held). Once this has been attained, the exercise programme can be progressed to include elements such as circuit weight-training, which should involve high repetition, low resistance, large muscle activity.

Further reading: Parr, R. B. (1996). Exercising when you're overweight. *Phys. Sports Med.*, **24**, issue No. 10.

93. Resistance exercise:

a. True b. True c. True d. True e. False

An isometric contraction is one in which the muscle develops tension but does not change length. An isotonic contraction is one in which the muscle shortens as it develops tension, and is the most familiar type of contraction, used during all lifting activities. An isokinetic contraction is defined as a contraction occurring at a constant speed over a range of motion at a variable resistance. Comparative studies of isokinetic, isotonic and isometric programmes have shown that there is a significantly greater increase in endurance and strength in individuals who engage in isokinetic rehabilitation programmes. Isokinetic training at slow speeds usually produce increases in strength only at slow movement speeds. Isokinetic training at fast speeds can produce increases in strength at all the speeds of movement; this training at fast speeds is also associated with increased muscle endurance at these faster speeds. The motivation is generally superior when an individual uses isotonic resistance exercise; this is thought to be due to the fact that it is itself a testing method of activity – that is, you either complete the task or you do not. Muscular endurance is developed more effectively through isotonic exercise rather than isometric, and the recovery from muscle fatigue is faster after isotonic exercise. Isotonic exercise also produces a more uniform development of strength. With the proliferation of fitness centres, isokinetic equipment has become more accessible; this method is now the resistance activity of choice when rehabilitating an individual following a musculoskeletal injury.

Further reading: Thistle, H. G., Hislop, H. J. and Moffroid, M. (1967). Isokinetic contraction: a new concept of resistive exercise. *Arch. Phys. Med. Rehab.*, **48**(6), 279–82.

Drugs, supplements and toxicology

94. Alcohol:

a. False b. True c. False d. True e. False

Eighty-five to ninety per cent of alcohol is metabolized in the liver by the enzyme alcohol dehydrogenase, and this occurs at the relatively slow fixed rate of 100 mg/kg per hour. This equates to a metabolic rate of 10 g per hour for a 100 kg man. There is a significant variation from person to person in the rate at which they metabolize alcohol. Exercise will not increase alcohol metabolism. Many recreational athletes believe that short-term ingestion of small amounts of alcohol enhances athletic performance. The American College of Sports Medicine conducted a comprehensive analysis of the science relating to the acute effects of alcohol in human performance in 1982. This showed that while the acute ingestion of alcohol had a deleterious effect on many cycle motor skills, it did not substantially influence physiological functions crucial to physical performance (VO_2 max, respiratory dynamics and cardiac function). The delayed effects of alcohol have also been considered, and it is suggested that a hangover will reduce aerobic performance due to its dehydrating effect on available carbohydrate and its effect on blood lactate levels. 85 per cent of alcohol is metabolized in the liver by the enzyme alcohol dehydrogenase. As the alcohol is being metabolized to aldehyde the substrate Nicotinamide Adenosine Dinucleotide (NAD) takes up a hydrogen ion (H+) resulting in an increase in NADH. This increases the NADH to NAD (oxidised NADH) ratio, which increases the production of lactic acid from pyruvate, increasing the lactate to pyruvate ratio. Increased levels of lactic acid will then limit activity during strenuous exercise. Beer is the choice of the majority of athletes who drink alcohol. A 330 ml (12 oz) can of beer contains approximately 150 calories and, of this, only 50 calories are in the form of carbohydrate. It is recommended that athletes consume 200–400 calories of carbohydrate within 2 hours of exercise, and then repeat this 2 hours later. To achieve this with beer alone, the athlete would have to drink up to eight cans of beer. This is both impractical and unwise, especially when a pint of fruit juice would meet the carbohydrate requirements. Beer is not therefore recommended as a fluid or nutritional replacement for the exercising athlete.

Further reading: O'Brien, C. P. (1993). Alcohol and sport. Impact of social drinking on recreational and competitive sports performance. *Sports Med.*, **15**(2), 71–7.

95. Erythropoietin:

a. True b. False c. False d. False e. True

Anecdotal evidence suggests that erythropoietin (EPO) is the athletic drug of abuse of the 1990s. EPO is used in clinical practice for patients with anaemias associated with chronic diseases such as renal failure. Erythropoietin creates red blood cells, thus boosting haemoglobin and haematocrit, and this increased haematocrit causes an increased viscosity in the blood.

Erythropoietin is banned as a blood doping offence, and is included in the IOC banned substance list. There is presently no IOC approved confirmatory procedure to detect this practice. Recombinant erythropoietin (rEPO) has a short half-life of approximately 4–6 hours when administered intravenously, and the detection of erythropoietin administration by determining abnormal concentrations in blood or urine is therefore difficult as the abuser can take steps to avoid giving a sample following administration of the drug.

This drug is abused by some athletes in an effort to improve their aerobic function, and they put themselves at risk of pulmonary embolism, clots, seizures or hypertensive encephalopathy. The International Olympic Committee and the national governing bodies of all Olympic sports have banned rEPO, and routine screening of haematocrit may suggest an abuser. However, defining an appropriate cut-off level for haematocrit is a fundamental problem; haematocrit levels greater than 0.52 in an otherwise healthy individual in the absence of a renal tumour or polycythaemia rubra vera would suggest an abuser. rEPO is identical to natural EPO immunologically and biologically, and is almost identical structurally. rEPO effects far outlast its detectability, and rEPO levels in the blood can return to baseline within days of injection. Routine haematocrit testing may be used as a screening method; however, it is not foolproof.

Further reading: Ramotar, J. E. (1990). Cyclist's death linked to erythropoietin. *Phys. Sports Med.*, **18**(8), 48-50.

96. Prohibited substances:

a. False b. True c. False d. True e. True

Performance-enhancing drugs are banned by the majority of sports' governing bodies. The International Olympic Council Medical Commission has taken the lead in defining and classifying banned substances. A performance-enhancing drug user is considered to be one who deliberately uses a drug in an attempt to gain an unfair advantage over fellow competitors. In 1986, the IOC produced a list of doping classes and methods. These are defined as follows:

1. Doping classes
   a. Stimulants
   b. Narcotic analgesics
   c. Anabolic steroids
   d. Beta-blockers
   e. Diuretics.
2. Doping methods
   a. Blood doping
   b. Pharmacological, chemical and physical manipulation.
3. Classes of drugs subject to certain restrictions
   a. Alcohol
   b. Local anaesthetics
   c. Corticosteroids.

The IOC lists examples of the drugs falling within each group. This list of drugs is not comprehensive, and includes the addendum that related compounds are also banned. It is important that physicians involved in sports medicine are aware of the up-to-date listing of doping classes and methods relating to particular sports as these vary from one sport to another.

97. Steroid injections:

a. True b. True c. False d. False e. False

The powerful anti-inflammatory effects of glucocortocoids have been known since 1949. The most potent form was that derived from hydrocortisone, the predominant glucocorticoid secreted in man.

Steroids cause their anti-inflammatory effects by a variety of means, none of which are clearly understood. They reduce the output of the chemical mediators of inflammation and inhibit the effect of the mediators on the vascular endothelium, resulting in a reduction in oedema and swelling. They also have effects on white blood cells; in particular, they reduce the activity of thymocytes, which are involved in the delayed hypersensitivity reaction. Prolonged use of steroids can disturb the metabolic activity of the body, resulting in a chemical Cushing's syndrome. In the sports setting, great care must be taken when injecting steroids. They have a catabolic effect on skeletal muscle, and a period of 10 days' rest following injection of a musculoskeletal structure is therefore essential.

Playing or taking activity during this period of time will increase the risk of the catabolic effect, and may ultimately cause a rupture of the injected structure. Many authors suggest that the injected area be treated with the RICE technique of first aid (see Answer 17) for 5–7 days following injection. Repeated joint injection increases the possibility of cortisone arthropathy; therefore, longer acting preparations such as trimcinolone hexacetonoide are indicated so that repeat injections are not necessary.

Further reading: Nirschl, R. P. and Sohel, J. (1981). Conservative treatment of tennis elbow. *Phys. Sports Med.*, **9**(6), 43–54.

98. Alcohol:

a. True b. False c. True d. False e. False

Alcohol is the drug most used by the athletic population. In general, 85–90 per cent of all athletes drink alcohol, and certain sports such as rugby union football traditionally have a higher incidence of alcohol use among players. The acute use of alcohol in the sports setting is associated with much morbidity and mortality. In particular, alcohol use on the water (either recreational or competitive) is significantly associated with drowning and near drowning episodes, and alcohol is a contributory factor in at least 60 per cent of all boating fatalities. A large proportion of those injured on the water have blood alcohol concentrations at a level that would preclude them from driving a motor vehicle. The acute use of alcohol has also been shown to reduce hand–eye co-ordination, and therefore operating a mechanically propelled vehicle or performing a high speed or motor activity requiring skill while under the influence of alcohol may increase the chances of accident. Alcohol ingestion may also be pro-arrhythmogenic in susceptible individuals, and is a causative factor for supraventricular tachycardias and lone atrial fibrillation. Its effect on the myocardium is ergolytic in that it decreases the pumping properties of the myocardium. Alcohol is also associated with an increased incidence of upper respiratory tract infections in running athletes.

Alcohol is subject to certain restrictions in competitive sports. It is a prohibited substance in some aiming events due to its ability to reduce tremor. Blood or breath alcohol levels may be requested in fencing and shooting events in the modern pentathlon; therefore, athletes competing in these events are advised to abstain from alcoholic beverages for at least 12 hours before the event.

99. Restricted drugs in sport:

a. False b. True c. False d. False e. False

The majority of major international events follow the recommendations laid down by the International Olympic Council regarding the use of pharmacological agents. These recommendations have divided prescribed drugs into two sections, Section 1 (banned drugs) and Section 2 (restricted drugs).

The restricted drugs are permissible only under certain conditions, and include injectable local anaesthetics, caffeine, alcohol, marijuana, beta-2 agonists and corticosteroids. Certain local anaesthetics are permitted, such as lidocaine and procaine, but cocaine is prohibited. The use of a local anaesthetic with a vasoconstrictor, such as epinephrine, is not permitted. The intravenous use of local anaesthetic is not permitted.

Corticosteroids are allowed for inhalation and topical use; they are also permitted for local or intra-articular injection. However, if a team doctor is considering an intra-articular or local steroid injection, he must give written notification to the International Olympic Council or competition medical director prior to treatment. The use of intravenous, intramuscular or oral corticosteroids is not permitted.

Caffeine is a prohibited substance if the blood level exceeds 12 mg/ml. With a normal daily caffeine intake this is unlikely; however, 10–12 mugs of percolated coffee may approach this level and the athlete should therefore be advised to maintain caffeine intake at a reasonable level.

The regularly prescribed beta-2 agonists terbutaline and salbutamol are permitted for inhalation; however, oral beta-2 agonists, and specifically fenoterol, are banned substances.

Alcohol is prohibited in certain aiming sports, such as fencing and shooting in the modern pentathlon. Its use should therefore be avoided for 12 hours prior to competition.

Marijuana is a commonly used street drug and is specifically banned by the National Collegiate Athletic Association (NCAA) in the United States of America. It is banned only for certain Olympic sports such as basketball and boxing; however, many governing sports bodies reserve the right to test athletes for marijuana at competitive events. The active ingredient in marijuana is delta-5-tetrahydro-cannabinol, and metabolites are detectable in the urine 4–10 days after smoking a marijuana cigarette. Passive inhalation of marijuana can also cause detectable levels in urine, and the thresholds used by governing bodies should therefore be sufficiently high to take this into account. Marijuana abuse can lead to impaired depth perception, which can be potentially hazardous in high speed or contact sports, where visualization of distance is important.

Further reading: Fuentes, R. J., Rosenberg, J. M. and Davis, A. (1996). *Athletic Drug Reference–96*. Glaxo Wellcome Inc. Clean Data Inc.

100. Mineral/iron supplementation:

a. False b. True c. False d. False e. True

Iron is a component of the red blood cells, and is involved in oxygen transportation. Reduced dietary intake has been observed in athletes who have to make weight, such as gymnasts and wrestlers, and in certain endurance-trained athletes, due to the mechanical trauma of exercise. The recommended daily intake for iron is 10 mg for men and 50 mg for women. The most appropriate way to ensure an adequate iron intake is to eat a balanced diet. Iron derived from animal foods is better absorbed than iron from plant foods. The iron in animal foods is described as haem iron, and eating a balanced diet that includes lean meat will give an adequate iron intake. Routine iron supplementation in the exercising athlete should be actively discouraged as this has many side effects, which can lead to morbidity and occasional mortality – anaphylaxis has been reported following iron supplementation use. A variety of symptoms, from nausea and constipation to cardiac arrhythmias, have been reported with the use of iron supplements, and any supplement should therefore be taken under medical supervision.

Further reading: Weight, L. M. (1993). Sports anaemia: does it exist? *Sports Med.*, **16**(1), 1–4.

101. Growth hormone:

a. True b. False c. True d. True e. False

Growth hormone (GH), growth hormone releasing factor (GHRF) and related somatotrophins are prohibited by both the International Olympic Committee and the National Collegiate Athletic Association in the United States of America. They are categorized as peptide hormones. In the 1980s, human growth hormone became more readily available for children with a growth hormone deficiency and short stature following the advances in synthetic production via recombinant DNA cloning. Abuse among athletes is thought to occur due to its lipolytic effect. There has been no evidence of increased skeletal muscle mass or strength in non-deficiency states; however, the effect on body fat appears to be sufficient for the abuse of this drug. There are many side effects associated with the abuse of human growth hormone, including gigantism and acromegaly, as well as the associated metabolic and endocrine disorders. There is also the suggestion that long-term abuse may be associated with leukaemia. Infection is also a problem with the abuse of human growth hormone. In the illicit market much of the human growth hormone is derived from cadavers, and may be contaminated by viruses such as the AIDS virus and CJD.

Further reading: Dipasquale, M. G. (1994). *Drugs in Sport*, **2**(4), 24–7.

102. Protein:

a. True b. False c. False d. False e. False

Protein is an essential daily nutrient for both the sedentary individual and the athlete. Guidelines suggest that between 12 and 30 per cent of the daily nutritional intake should be in the form of protein. The actual daily intake can be calculated per kg or pound of body weight per day. The daily recommended intake for a sedentary adult is 0.9 g of protein per kg per day; competitive adult athletes should consume approximately 1.8 g of protein per kg of body weight per day, and growing teenagers should consume upwards of 2.2 g per kg body weight per day. Many athletes follow a 'fad'-type dietary regimen and survive on a low saturated fat diet. Not only is protein sacrificed in this type of diet, but also iron and zinc, both essential daily nutrients. Most vegetarian diets can supply sufficient protein if individuals ensure that they eat a variety of foods that contain sufficient essential amino acids, such as beans and rice tofu.

Further reading: Lemon, P. W., Tarnopolsky, M. A. and MacDougall, J. D. (1992). Protein requirements and muscle mass–strength changes during intensive training in novice body builders. *J. Appl. Physiol.*, **73**(2), 767–75.

103. Ergolytic drugs:

a. True b. True c. False d. True e. True

Ergolytic drugs are described as pharmacological agents that can impair athletic performance and may contribute to fatigue. Examples of ergolytic drugs include tobacco, marijuana and alcohol. Marijuana curbs exercise performance by increasing resting heart rates. The nicotine in tobacco raises heart rates and blood pressure, resulting in an increased pulse pressure per unit of work. Cardiac stroke, output and heart rate are all negatively affected by chronic use of tobacco. The use of these recreational drugs should therefore be discouraged among the athletic population, as they affect physiological performance. The Beta blocker used to treat hypertension, Propranolol, is also an ergolytic agent for the following reasons:

1. It reduces tidal volume during heavy exercise
2. It attenuates the exercise-induced rise in heart rate and blood pressure
3. It alters skin blood flow and sweat rates and affects core temperature.

It should therefore be discouraged among the athletic population.

Further reading: Sutton, J. R. (1978). Hormonal and metabolic responses to exercise in subjects of high and low work capacities. *Medicine and Science in Sports*, **10**, 1-6.

104. Chromium:

a. True b. True c. True d. True

Chromium is a naturally occurring mineral. It is involved in normal glucose metabolism, insulin and fatty acid metabolism and in muscle. It is found in shellfish; however, chromium can easily be destroyed by food processing and cooking. The recommended daily intake of chromium is 50–200 mg in the sedentary population. It is suggested that the exercising athlete requires greater levels of chromium, as the increased insulin metabolism associated with exercise puts a greater demand on the body's chromium stores. The harder the exercise, the greater the chromium use. Trivalent chromium is suggested to be a glucose tolerance factor or a facilitator of normal glucose metabolism; this agent is not toxic, even in very large doses. Hexavalent chromium, however, is highly toxic, and is known to be carcinogenic. Chromium in the form of chromium picolinate is a mineral supplement widely used by the exercising athletic population. Upwards of 92 per cent of all exercising American female athletes regularly take vitamins and mineral supplementation. The chromium use by the athletic population is due to the suggested increase in insulin metabolism caused by exercise, which increases the body's chromium requirements. Research has indicated significant loss on training days as opposed to non-training days. Sources of chromium include inorganic forms such as chromium chloride; however, the biological activity of inorganic chromium is low.

Newer, more biologically active formulations have been developed, and the most commonly encountered variety is chromium picolinate, which was developed in Minnesota. This formulation has a significantly better absorption than the inorganic chromiums. Research among the athletic population has shown reductions in body fat percentage and increases in lean body mass in athletes who are supplemented with this mineral when compared to controls. Presently this mineral supplement is not banned by any of the regulating sports authorities. Its use, however, is in its infancy, and care with dosing and use should therefore be advised because its long-term effects have as yet not been fully established. Great care should be taken in using these supplements, and discussion of all nutrient supplementation should be encouraged between the athlete and the doctor because an athlete will often use an inappropriate formulation or dosage in an effort to gain a legal advantage over fellow competitors.

Further reading: Anderson, R. A., Bryden, N. A. and Polansky, M. M. (1988). Exercise effects on chromium excretion of trained and untrained men consuming a constant diet. *J. Appl. Physiol.*, **64**(1), 249-52.

105. Zinc:

a. True b. False c. False d. True e. False

Zinc is a component of many of the body's enzymes. Normal zinc metabolism is essential for the proper functioning of the immune system and of the reproductive system in the male, as zinc is essential for normal testosterone levels and sperm counts. The recommended daily intake of zinc is 15 mg; however, research has shown that the average 2850 calorie American diet falls short of this recommended daily allowance by over 10 per cent. Certain athletes may have an increased demand for zinc due to greater loss from red cell haemolysis (see Answer 5 on athletic anaemia) and from losses in sweat. There may also be an increased demand for zinc by the exercising individual due to the increased fatty acid metabolism. There is research that suggests that exercise of itself may reduce the zinc status. In a similar way to iron deficiency, sports in which making weight is an integral component have a particular susceptibility to zinc deficiency due to an inadequate dietary intake (wrestling, gymnastics and dance). Distance runners also have an increased susceptibility to zinc deficiency due to foot strike haemolysis and blood loss from the bowel and bladder. Zinc toxicity occurs at a relatively low level, and is reported at an intake of 500 mg/day; therefore, as with all supplementations, the athlete has to be carefully tutored and advised regarding supplementation with this potentially hazardous mineral.

Further reading: Couzy, F., Lafargue, P. and Guezennec, C. Y. (1990). Zinc metabolism in the athlete; influence of training, nutrition and other factors. *Int. J. Sports Med.*, **11**, 263–6.

106. Antioxidants:

a. False b. True c. True d. False e. True

Muscle power is generated by the conversion of adenosine triphosphate (ATP) into energy. This can occur aerobically or anaerobically. ATP is generated aerobically by two processes:

1. Tetravalent reduction of oxygen with cytochrome C oxidase
2. Univalent reduction of oxygen.

The second pathway produces free radicals during exercise; namely, superoxide free radicals, hydroperoxide free radicals and hydroxyl free radicals. These free radicals increase during exercise, and are associated with muscle damage after exercise. The hydroxyl free radicals continue to cause injury. the hydroxyl free radicals react with the fat in the muscle cell membranes in a process called lipid peroxidation; the damaged fats also become free radicals called peroxyl radicals. These do further tissue damage and produce further free radicals, which can result in an inflammatory chain reaction that may persist for many hours after exercise. Neutrophils are then released to mop up the dead muscle cells. Following this, further free radicals are released. The net result is a significant free radical release after intense exercise, which leaves the body stiff, sore and unable to exercise properly for up to 5 days.
Antioxidants are the body's defence mechanism against the free radicals. There are three main antioxidants:

a. Catalase, this neutralizes hydrogen peroxides
b. Superoxide dismutase (SOD), which destroys superoxide radicals
c. Glutathione peroxidase, which detoxifies peroxides.

Catalase and superoxide dismutase are synthesized endogenously, and oral supplementation does not alter serum levels as they are destroyed by the digestive process. The glutathione system, however, can be manipulated. Animal studies have shown that intensive exercise can reduce muscle glutathione levels. It is postulated that glutathione levels can be increased by supplementing with the amino acids and, in particular, cysteine, which make up glutathione. Many athletes supplement with N-acetyl cysteine in an effort to increase serum glutathione levels. This is at best an experimental strategy, with potential side-effects. Vitamin C, vitamin E, selenium and coenzyme Q10 are also considered to have antioxidant properties. Vitamin E in particular has attained much public notoriety in the recent years as an antioxidant. It is thought to break the lipid peroxidation chain reaction by absorbing free radicals to form tocopherol and tocopheroxyl radicals. These tocopheroxyl radicals are neutralized by vitamin C, with subsequent regeneration of vitamin E. The recommended daily intake of vitamin E is 10 mg/day, although it is suggested that the athletic requirement may be greater. Research to date, however, has indicated that oral vitamin E supplementation results in few side effects, even when the normal daily recommended allowance is exceeded. Selenium is also involved in an antioxidant effect. It is suggested that it acts synergistically with vitamin E and forms active sites for glutathione activity on lipid peroxide radicals. This mineral, however, can be extremely toxic, and should be used with great care. The use of antioxidants in the athletic population is in its infancy, and great care and supervision is therefore essential when employing these agents. In particular, selenium can become very toxic at levels above 800 mg/day and N-acetyl cysteine is associated with the development of kidney stones if it is not used in association with vitamin C.

Further reading: Bendich, A. and Machlin, F. J. (1988). Safety of oral intake of vitamin E. *Am. J. Clin. Nutr.* **48**, 612–19.

107. Carbohydrates:

a. True b. True c. True d. False e. False

Carbohydrates serve a number of important functions in the body:

1. They are essential for the normal functioning of the central nervous system (CNS). Blood sugar is the predominant fuel for the brain; however, during starvation, metabolic adaptation can occur and after 8 days the brain is able to use a relatively large amount of fat for its fuel requirements.
2. Carbohydrate acts as the main energy fuel for muscular contraction. Adequate dietary carbohydrate is required to maintain the body's glycogen stores. It is suggested that active people should take upwards of 60 per cent of their daily calorific intake in the form of carbohydrates. These

should be predominantly of the complex carbohydrate variety. If too few carbohydrates are ingested, then glucose is attained from glycogen breakdown. If excess carbohydrates are absorbed, these are converted to muscle glycogen. Once glycogen capacity has been reached, the excess carbohydrate is converted into fat stores.

3. Carbohydrate also has a protein-sparing effect. If carbohydrate reserves are reduced, protein gluconeogenesis occurs to increase blood sugar. This may occur during starvation or prolonged endurance activity. If carbohydrate intake is adequate, then this tissue protein is spared from gluconeogenesis.
4. Carbohydrate also has to be available to facilitate normal fat metabolism. If carbohydrate metabolism is reduced, fat mobilization and metabolism increases to beyond the capacity of the body to metabolize it adequately. This results in incomplete fat metabolism, and the accumulation of ketone bodies and acidosis.

Further reading: Fielding, R. A. (1985). Effects of carbohydrate feeding, frequencies and dosage on muscle glycogen use during exercise. *Med. Sci. Sports Exer.*, **17**, 472.

108. Melatonin:

a. True b. True c. False d. False e. False

Melatonin is a hormone that is secreted by the pineal gland. Since 1995, this hormone has been used as an over-the-counter dietary supplement. It is used to treat a variety of medical ailments; however, there is very little scientific data to back up many of the claims relating to its use. Research has indicated that it can help individuals with mild to moderate sleep disorders, and it can also be helpful in fighting jet lag. It is classified as a dietary supplement, and therefore does not come under the regulation of the Food and Drug Administration Standards. Care would be advised when using this supplement.

109. The phosphagens:

a. True b. True c. True d. True e. True

Phosphocreatine and ATP are energy-rich phosphate compounds that are stored in muscle cells. The total musculature stores of both ATP and phosphocreatine are very small; only about 0.3 mol in females and 0.6 mol in males. The amount of energy obtained from this system is limited, and these phosphagen stores would probably be empty by the end of a 100–200 m sprint. The phosphagen system, however, is important due to the rapid availability of energy. It is the energy system used for physical activity such as kicking, jumping, swinging and sprinting. When ATP is broken down during musculature contraction, it is rapidly reformed by the energy liberated during the breakdown of phosphocreatine.

Anatomy

110. The axillary nerve:

a. False b. True c. True d. False e. True

The axillary nerve arises off the posterior cord of the brachial plexus. It sends a motor supply to the deltoid and the teres minor muscles, and supplies sensation to the upper outer forearm region referred to as the 'Boy Scout patch' area. The axillary nerve can be damaged following dislocation of the shoulder joint, as the nerve has a relatively fixed origin off the brachial plexus and is vulnerable to a stretch injury in the quadrilateral space. It can also be injured by direct trauma to the shoulder area. The normal pattern of injury is a neuropathic lesion, and it is suggested that there is subclinical involvement of the axillary nerve in up to 30 per cent of anterior dislocations. The patient may present with numbness in the upper outer shoulder or an inability to abduct the shoulder due to weakness of the deltoid muscle. Electromyography of the deltoid muscle will show evidence of denervation 3–4 weeks post-injury. These denervation potentials may persist for up to 1 year after the event; however, in the majority of cases the patient will recover fully over 2–3 months. Isokinetic dynamometry can be a useful aid in deciding when to return the individual to activity. It is suggested that an abduction value approaching 90 per cent of that on the contralateral side is an acceptable level for return to activity.

Further reading: Blom, S. and Dahlback, L. O. (1970). Nerve injuries in dislocations of the shoulder joint and fractures of the neck of humerus. *Acta. Chir. Scand.*, **136**(6), 461-6.

111. Fracture at the base of the 5th metatarsal:

a. False b. True c. True d. True

An inversional ankle injury can result in pathology remote from the ankle joint, and a fracture at the base of the 5th metatarsal is such an injury. It results from an avulsion of the insertion of the peroneus brevis tendon. The fracture occurs due to a forced inversional injury, which results in avulsion of the insertion of the tendon. Clinical examination of the foot as well as the ankle following inversional injuries is essential to rule out this common injury. Pain is usually elicited at the base of the 5th metatarsal on palpation. Positive X-rays usually show a fracture line that is transverse to the long axis of the metatarsal. In younger individuals this has to be differentiated from a normal unfused apophysis; in these instances the apophysis usually lies longitudinal to the long axis of the metatarsal, and therefore should not be misinterpreted as a fracture.

112. Scaphoid fractures:

a. False b. False c. True d. True e. True

Ninety per cent of carpal bone fractures are through the scaphoid bone. Clinically, the patient may give a history of falling on an outstretched hand and often describes generalized wrist pain. Clinical examination will often but not always identify the anatomical snuffbox tenderness. As scaphoid fractures are often very difficult to demonstrate, four scaphoid views should be ordered at X-ray. Eighty per cent of fractures are at the waist of the scaphoid, 10 per cent at the proximal pole and a further 10 per cent at the distal pole. Fractures across the waist and proximal pole compromise the blood supply of the proximal fragment and, if treatment is inappropriate or incorrect, non-union and avascular necrosis of the bone may result. Proximal pole injuries carry the greatest risk of avascular necrosis, with waist injuries carrying a slightly lesser risk. Distal pole fractures do not carry any risk of avascular necrosis, as the blood supply is not compromised. Initial scaphoid X-rays may not identify the fracture site, and in many centres the patient is treated prophylactically in a scaphoid cast despite the absence of a fracture on the initial X-rays. The patient should be reviewed 1–2 weeks later, and radiology repeated. Many scaphoid fractures are not detectable until this time, but resorption of the bone around the fracture will have occurred and the majority of fractures may be visible at this stage. Further radiological investigations such as three-phase bone scanning may be required in cases where a fracture is not detectable on X-ray but the clinical signs suggest its presence.

113. Acromioclavicular joint subluxation:

a. True b. True c. True d. False e. True

Acromioclavicular joint injuries are very common among those participating in 'falling' sports such as equestrianism, skiing and rugby union football. The history of acromioclavicular joint injury is usually that of a fall onto the point of the shoulder, generally accompanied by acute pain at the upper margin of the shoulder joint. Clinical examination may reveal tenderness at the level of the posterior acromioclavicular joint. Shoulder abduction usually causes further pain at a level of 120° of abduction. Shoulder adduction, with a flexed elbow across the chest, also causes local pain. Occasionally the accessory nerve may be injured, and sensory testing of the outer upper shoulder and arm is therefore essential to identify any sensory abnormality in the distribution of the axillary nerve. Radiology is helpful in grading acromioclavicular subluxations (1–4). The antero-posterior view is usually the most helpful; the width of the normal acromioclavicular joint is variable, but it is usually less than 10 mm in adults. However, enlargement above this level should not be considered in isolation, but rather in comparison to the contralateral acromioclavicular joint. In a healthy acromioclavicular joint, the inferior surface of the acromion and the clavicle should be in a straight line; subluxation of the joint is detected by a break in this line. Weight-bearing views of the right and left side can be helpful in equivocal cases. This is also helpful in grading the lesion. Grade 4 acromioclavicular joint subluxations usually signify disruption of the coraco-acromial ligaments, and significant widening and separation is noted on AP radiology. This frequently requires surgical intervention.

114. Vastus medialis muscle:

a. False b. False c. False d. True e. True

The vastus medialis is part of the quadriceps complex; it can be located at the distal 20 per cent of the medial tie, and at this level the oblique fibres of the vastus medialis muscle are angled at nearly 45° towards the patella. The function of this muscle is to counteract the pull of the lateral quadriceps muscles, and it is therefore an essential stabilizer of the patellofemoral joint. Weakness of the vastus medialis oblique fibres is associated with patellofemoral syndrome. In individuals who have an increased Q angle, the function of this muscle is essential to prevent symptoms of patellofemoral syndrome. The vastus medialis muscle receives its nerve supply from the femoral nerve, with a root innervation at L2, 3, 4. A disc lesion can therefore occasionally cause local leg pain and atrophy of the muscles in the myotomal distribution.

115. The supraspinatus muscle:

a. False b. False c. True d. False e. False

The supraspinatus muscle is part of the rotator cuff complex. The muscle is located at the medial third of the scapular spine, where it receives its origin. It is inserted into the greater tuberosity of the humerus via the supraspinatus tendon. This tendon is commonly involved in an overuse tendonopathy, which is often observed in racket sports players. The supraspinatus muscle receives its innervation in combination with the infraspinatus muscle by the suprascapular nerve. This nerve is liable to damage at the suprascapular notch following direct trauma, and may result in atrophy and dysfunction of both muscles. More commonly in the sporting arena, this muscle may become damaged following an upper trunk brachial plexus injury that may occur as a consequence of a stinger or burner type injury. In these instances, the supraspinatus, infraspinatus, deltoid and biceps are usually the affected muscles. Following direct trauma to the shoulder or neck, the athlete may complain of a burning dysaesthesia affecting the lateral aspect of the thumb and weakness in shoulder motion. Shoulder abduction (supraspinatus and deltoid) elbow flexion (biceps) and shoulder external rotation (infraspinatus) are usually affected.

Neurophysiological assessment and follow-up is essential to ensure an appropriate recovery prior to returning to a contact sport.

116. The adductor longus:

a. False b. False c. True d. True e. True

The adductor longus muscle takes its origin from the pubic tubercle. It is inserted into the linea sprea between the adductor magnus and the vastus medialis. It adducts the lower limb, and receives its nerve supply from the obturator nerve, receiving its root supply from the anterior divisions of the lumbar plexus (L2, 3, 4). This muscle can therefore be compromised by injury to the obturator nerve in L2, 3, 4 root lesions and in lumbar plexus lesions involving the anterior divisions. It is often injured in the sporting community by those athletes who frequently twist and turn, and is commonly seen in rugby scrum-halves, soccer midfielders and hockey players. The patient may complain of generalized pubic pain. Careful palpation of the pubis may reveal local tenderness at the pubic tubercle, which may be exacerbated by both abduction and adduction.

Cardiology and sport

117. Lone atrial fibrillation:

a. False b. False c. False d. True e. False

Lone atrial fibrillation is defined as fibrillation occurring in the absence of rheumatic valve disease or associated medical conditions which provoke atrial fibrillation, such as thyroid disease. The atrial fibrillation is usually provoked by an exogenous triggering factor such as ingestion of caffeine, alcohol and ice cream in association with activity. Similarly, exercise in cold water has also been shown to provoke atrial fibrillation. Treatment involves avoiding the triggering factor. Should atrial fibrillation occur despite such avoidance, then digoxin, beta-blockers or Class 1 anti-arrhythmic agents may be used. Atrial fibrillation is not a benign condition, and is associated with over 75 000 strokes per year in North America. Therefore, anticoagulant agents are often used. While lone atrial fibrillation does not preclude an individual from vigorous athletic activity, patients on anticoagulant medication should avoid contact sports.

Further reading: Brand, F. N., Abbott, R. D. and Cannil, W. B. (1985). Characteristics and prognosis of lone atrial fibrillation: 30 year follow-up in the Framingham study. *JAMA*, **254**(24), 3449-53.

118. Common rhythm disturbances:

a. True b. False c. True d. True e. True

Rhythm disturbances are commonly seen in the athletic population. The most common abnormality is sinus bradycardia, with some studies suggesting a prevalence exceeding 50 per cent. The degree of bradycardia correlates with the intensity of the training. The cause of the bradycardia is suggested to be that of exercise vagal predominance, referred to as vagotonia. This is thought to represent either an increase in vagal tone or a decrease in sympathetic tone. Atrioventricular block is occasionally seen in the athletic population. The AV block is usually first degree block, which is detected in upwards of 37 per cent of resting ECGs in the athletic population. Second degree block (Mobitz type 1) is related to training, and does not appear to have any association with evolving cardiac disease. Mobitz type 2 and third degree heart block are rarely seen in the athletic population. Junctional rhythms are also reported, and certain studies suggest a prevalence of up to 20 per cent in athletes.

119. Athletic heart syndrome:

a. False b. True c. True d. False e. True

Alterations in repolarization are the predominant manifestation of the training effects on the electrocardiogram. SE segment and T wave changes are the most commonly seen. The changes observed in the athletic heart syndrome include increased P wave amplitude, left ventricular hypertrophy and, less frequently, right ventricular hypertrophy. The repolarization changes include SE segment elevation, T wave inversion in the lateral precordial, tall peaked T waves and, occasionally, byphasic T waves in leads V3 to V6. The SE segment elevation varies but, in general, the more highly trained the athletes, the more likely it is to be present.

Further reading: Zeppilli, P., Pirami, M. M. and Sassara, F. (1981). Ventricular repolarization disturbances in athletes. Standardization of terminology, ethipathogenic spectrum and pathophysiological mechanism. *J. Sports Med. Phys. Fit.*, **21**(4), 322–35.

120. Marfan's syndrome:

a. True b. True c. True d. True e. True

Marfan's syndrome is a potentially fatal condition, due to cystic medial necrosis of the aorta. It is more commonly seen in the athletic population due to the large stature of these individuals. Because of the potentially fatal consequences of this condition in association with exercise, it is suggested that all men over 190 cm (~ 6 ft 4 in) and all women over 175 cm (~ 5 ft 10 in) in height who have two of the following criteria be screened with slit lamp examination and electrocardiogram:

1. Family history of Marfan's syndrome
2. Arm span greater than height
3. Antero-thoracic deformity
4. Kypho-scoliosis
5. Cardiac murmur or mid-systolic click
6. Ectopic lens
7. Myopia

8. Upper to lower body ratio more than one standard deviation below the mean.

121. Hypertrophic cardiomyopathy in the athletic population:

a. True b. True c. True d. True e. True

Sudden death among the athletic population remains a relatively rare but significant risk of participation in sport, and the major cause of sudden death in the sports setting is that of cardiac disease. In the older athlete, this is usually caused by coronary artery disease. In the younger population, structural abnormalities are the major cause. Hypertrophic cardiomyopathy is far and away the most common structural abnormality identified in younger individuals who die while exercising. During a pre-participation examination clinical signs associated with hypertrophic cardiomyopathy can be elicited, and this may be the only opportunity to identify an athlete with a potentially fatal condition. The majority of the findings are associated with ventricular outflow obstruction. The pulse is usually jerky but sustained; this is caused by the powerful ventricular contraction and mitral regurgitation producing a rapid initial upstroke, followed by a second small sustained component caused by the flow through the systolic outflow obstruction. Palpation of the precordium usually identifies a double apical impulse. This is caused by the palpable atrial filling thrust, followed by the forceful impulse of the left ventricular hypertrophy. A third heart sound can be heard, and is thought to correspond with a sudden halt in the rapid ventricular filling. A fourth heart sound may also be heard; a late systolic murmur can be heard due to the outflow tract obstruction and a concomitant mitral regurgitation.

Further reading: McKenna, D., Gehrakej, W. J. and Goodwin, J. F. (1979). Diagnosis of obstructive hypertrophic cardiomyopathy: is echocardiography of value? *Br. Heart. J.*, **41**, 379.

122. Aortic insufficiency and exercise:

a. True b. False c. True d. False e. False

Cardiac murmurs can be detected in 30–85 per cent of athletes who participate in dynamic sports. History and cardiovascular examination remains the mainstay of picking up cardiac abnormalities. Aortic regurgitation can often be asymptomatic, and may be picked up as an incidental finding on a pre-participation examination. Aortic insufficiency can remain asymptomatic for long periods in an athlete, as exercise decreases the peripheral vascular resistance and diastolic filling time with a resultant decrease in regurgitant volume. There is also an increased forward flow through the aortic valve with exercise. Prolonged exposure to high regurgitant volumes, however, can result in cardiac dilatation and left ventricular failure. This may present with a sudden onset of symptoms of congestive heart failure, angina or sudden death. The 26th Bethesda Conference recommended that athletes with aortic regurgitation should not participate in any competitive sport if they have severe aortic regurgitation, or if they have moderate regurgitation and are symptomatic. Aortic regurgitation is a possibly life-threatening condition that may affect the athletic population; therefore, all pre-participation examinations should include a careful auscultation of the precordium. The detection of a systolic murmur requires further evaluation by electrocardiogram, chest X-ray, echocardiogram or, occasionally, a Muga scan (an exercise multiple gated acquisition scan). This latter scan will observe the resting left ventricular ejection fraction and also the ejection fraction with exercise. Treatment may involve a valve replacement. Research has shown a favourable outcome with prosthetic valve use, and no particular prosthetic valve dysfunction or increased haemolysis has been noticed with vigorous exercise. However, the decision regarding clearance for returning to competitive play following valve replacement has to be taken on a patient-by-patient basis.

Further reading: The 26th Bethesda Conference (1994). Recommendations for determining eligibility for competition in athletes with cardiovascular abnormalities, January 6–7, 1994. *J. & Coll. Cardiol.*, **24**(4), 845–99.

Exercise physiology

123. Functional aerobic impairment:

a. True b. True c. True d. True e. False

The functional capacity is described as the maximum oxygen uptake. It can be predicted from submaximal exercise tests, and values can be expressed either in absolute or rate-relative units. Predicted maximal aerobic power reflects the ability of an individual to perform external work. Functional capacity can be reduced by many clinical conditions. Factors that affect maximum heart rate, maximum stroke volume, arterial oxygen content and mixed venous oxygen content can all reduce the functional capacity. The functional aerobic impairment is a concept that was designed to quantify the degree of disability resulting from clinical conditions. The percentage FAI is a value derived from a predicted VO_2 max minus the observed VO_2 max divided by the predicted VO_2 max. It is essentially the percentage by which an individual's functional capacity falls below that expected for his or her age, sex and conditioning. FAI can be described according to a quantitative scale, where levels above 68 per cent indicate extreme impairment and levels between 0 per cent and 26 per cent show no significant functional aerobic impairment. Negative values for FAI indicate that functional capacity is above average.

Further reading: Bruce, R. A., Kusumi, F. and Hosmer, D. (1973). Maximal oxygen intake and homographic assessment of functional aerobic impairment in cardiovascular disease. *Am. Heart J.*, **85**(4), 546–62.

124. Second wind:

a. True b. True c. True d. False e. True

'Second wind' is described as the sudden easing of dyspnoea during heavy exercise. It is suggested that the second wind is related to improved contractility of the diaphragm due to increased circulating catecholamines and changes in diaphragmatic blood flow. There are no changes observed in the accessory muscles of respiration, recruitment, chest configuration or in diaphragmatic pressures.

Further reading: Fragoso, C. V. and Systrom, D. M. (1991). The

Respiratory System. In *Sports Medicine* (R. H. Strauss, ed.), 2nd edn. W. B. Saunders.

125. Muscle contractions:

a. True b. False c. False d. True e. True

Muscle contractions can be classified as concentric, which is muscle length shortening while developing tension, or eccentric, which is muscle lengthening while developing tension. An isometric muscle contraction results in the muscle developing tension, but it does not change in length. An isotonic muscle contraction results in the muscle shortening while developing tension; an example of this would be the biceps muscle during a barbell elbow flexion exercise. An isokinetic muscle contraction results in the muscle shortening while developing maximal tension throughout the full range of movement; this occurs at a constant speed. Isokinetic muscle contractions occur at a constant speed and a variable resistance, whereas isotonic muscle contractions occur at a variable speed with a constant resistance.

126. Fast twitch motor units:

a. True b. False c. False d. True e. True

Fast twitch muscle fibres are characterized by a fast contraction time, high anaerobic capacity and low aerobic capacity, all making the fibre suited for high power output activities. They usually have a low capillary density and a high force of contraction, but fatigue rapidly. In general, endurance athletes have a predominance of slow twitch fibres, whereas non-endurance athletes such as sprinters, shot putters and weight-lifters have a higher percentage of fast twitch fibres. However, it should be noted that there is a very large variation in fibre types among all athletic groups, and it is suggested that the fibre type may be a determinant in the selection of the athlete's sport.

Further reading: Burke, E. R., Cerney, F., Costill, D. and Fink, W. (1977). Characteristics of skeletal muscle in competitive cyclists. *Med. Sci. Sports*, **9**(2), 109–112.

127. Sleep and exercise:

a. True b. True c. True d. False e. False

Insomnia is one of the cardinal signs of the over-training syndrome. The other three signs are:

1. Elevation in resting daily heart rate by 8 beats per minute
2. Reduction in stable body weight by more than 1.5 kg (~ 3 lb)
3. Alteration in immunity, with particular elevations of ESR, lymphocytes, monocytes and eosinophils in the absence of infection.

Insomnia or sleep disturbance is often difficult to identify in the athlete suffering from the over-training syndrome. Research has indicated that the over-training syndrome occurs primarily because of insufficient rest. Athletes should get 7–9½ hours of sleep a night. Athletes who train more than once a day should also try and have a catnap of 45 minutes during the day before the second training session. If an athlete is suffering from the over-training syndrome, it is not adequate to merely increase the nightly sleeping period. Sleeping should be increased to up to 9 hours per night; however, this should also be accompanied by alterations in the diet, including reducing protein intake to 15 per cent and increasing carbohydrate to greater than 70 per cent of the total calorie intake. Training should also be cut back, with complete cessation for a period of 1–2 weeks. The athlete can then return to activity at a lower frequency, duration and intensity, and slowly build up again to the previous training level.

Further reading: Fry, R. W., Morton, A. R. and Keast, D. (1991). Over-training in athletes. *Sports Med.*, **12**(1), 32–65.

128. Aerobic and anaerobic energy system contributions during sporting activities:

a. True b. True c. False d. True e. True

The aerobic and anaerobic energy systems contribute at least some ATP during performance of the activity. One system usually contributes more during a given activity, and athletes in particular sports therefore often have a selectively developed energy system. Often athletes with a particular genetic make-up self-select a suitable sport. Rapid one-off activities such as a golf and tennis swing derive all their energy from the anaerobic system, with no contribution whatsoever from the aerobic system. In a similar way, basketball and baseball players and wrestlers gain almost 90 per cent of their energy from the anaerobic system. Participants in longer distance activities such as jogging and marathon running take all their energy from the aerobic system initially. The 10 000 m skaters take 90 per cent of their energy from the aerobic system. Boxers, 1500 m skaters and 200 m swimmers have a 50/50 split of the two energy systems. Rowers in the 2000 m event have a 60/40 split in favour of the aerobic system.

Further reading: Fox, E. L. (ed.) (1992). Sports Activities and the Energy Continuum. In *Sports Physiology*. Holt-Saunders.

129. Sleep:

a. True b. True c. False d. True e. False

Sleep duration is associated with all causes of mortality. In a large study of males and females of 45 years or older, those who reported sleeping more than 10 hours or fewer than 5 hours per night had an elevated mortality risk. Those who reported sleeping about 7 hours per night had the lowest death rate. This association between sleep duration and mortality has been subsequently confirmed by other research. Exercise has been shown to reduce the resting sympathetic nerve activity, and this is postulated to have a direct effect on mortality. The risk of an acute coronary event is highest in the morning, just after wakening from sleep. Rapid eye movement sleep dominates the last third of the sleep period, and this time is dominated by a profound increase in the sympathetic nerve activity. It is suggested that this increased sympathetic activity during rapid eye movement sleep may initiate platelet aggregation, plaque rupture or coronary vasospasm, thus acting as a trigger for a cardiac event that may occur after wakening. Epidemiological studies have shown that exercise is helpful in promoting sleep, and may also improve the quality of sleep. Exercise may have a role in down-regulating sympathetic activity during sleep and, in this way, may have a role to play in acute cardiac events after awakening.

Further reading: Somers, V. K., Dyken, M. E. and Mark, A. L. (1993). Sympathetic nerve activity during sleep in normal subjects. *N. Engl. J. Med.*, **328**, 303–7.

130. Physiological assessment:

a. False b. True c. False d. True e. False

Physiological assessment has become part and parcel of all team sports.

Group or field testing has become particularly popular, as large groups of individuals may be tested together without recourse to expensive physiological equipment. Aerobic capacities can be tested by performance tests such as the Kline 1-mile walk test, the Lusbera shuttle run test and the Cooper's 12-minute run/walk test. The Kline and Cooper's tests are particularly useful in assessing large groups of participants. The Kline test formulates an arithmetic calculation based on the finishing heart rate, body weight and time taken to complete the 1-minute walk test. From these parameters, an estimation of the maximum oxygen uptake can be calculated. In a similar way, the Cooper's 12-minute run test calculates a maximum oxygen uptake from a normogram. The initial research investigated a large group of American airforce recruits. These individuals underwent a 12-minute run on a track, and the distance travelled by each individual was measured. Following this, they underwent a formal Douglas bag VO_2 max assessment. A correlation between the distance travelled by recruits in 12 minutes and their VO_2 max was therefore established, and a correlation between distance travelled and VO_2 max was established. This particular method for assessing VO_2 max is very common among the rugby playing population, and was also used to assess the soccer referees prior to the recent world cup in the United States of America. Anaerobic power output can also be assessed by performance tests. The Sergeant jump is probably the most popular. This involves a standing jump, the height of the jump relating to a power output. Specific watt power outputs can be established from a Bosco Ergo jump test. This calculates the power output during a sequence of standing jumps over a 15- or 45- second period. The most popular field test of anaerobic power output in the United States of America is the 40-yard dash. This particular test is performed by American football teams in spring training, and is considered to be a significant benchmark – many individuals who fall short of the acceptable standard are jettisoned from the American football team. Each of these anaerobic performance tests is activity specific, and there is therefore poor correlation of power outputs between each test. For this reason, it is essential to pick a test that is specific to the particular sporting activity that the tested individuals engage in. For example, basketball players would perform extremely well at the jump test, but not at the 40-yard dash; the reverse may be true of American football players.

Further reading: Bal Monte, A. (1988). Exercise testing and ergometers. In *The Olympic Book of Sports Medicine* (A. Dirix, J. J. Knuttgen and K. Tittel, eds). Blackwell Science.

131. Ozone and exercise:

a. True b. True c. False d. True e. True

Ozone is an urban air pollutant caused by the action of sunlight on motor vehicle and industrial emissions. Ozone is a potent airway irritant, and levels of 0.18 ppm are regularly observed in major metropolitan areas. Elevated atmospheric ozone levels have been shown to impair lung function and exercise performance. Typical symptoms of ozone exposure include cough, substernal pain after taking a deep breath and a feeling of chest tightness, which may mimic a cardiac episode. Exercise performance can be significantly altered even at low levels of ozone concentration (0.12 ppm). In particular, reduction in force FEV1 (forced expiratory volume in 1 second) of the order of 6 per cent has been observed at ozone concentration of 0.12 ppm, escalating to a reduction of FEV1 of 22 per cent at concentrations of 0.20 ppm. Levels as low as 0.08 ppm have also been shown to induce small changes in lung function. Recovery from ozone-induced lung function and respiratory symptoms usually occurs within hours.

$V0_2$ max has been found to be significantly decreased following two hours of intermittent exposure to 0.75 ppm of ozone. This is probably due to the reduced alveolar air exchange with subsequent reduction in oxygen transfer. Healthy young adults are more affected by ozone exposure than healthy older adults, and cardiac patients who are exposed to ozone during moderate exercise showed no particular alterations in onset of cardiovascular symptoms or signs, suggesting that ozone had no direct effect on the cardiovascular system.

Further reading: Superko, H. R., Adams, W. C. and Daly, P. W. (1984). Effects of ozone inhalation during exercise on selected patients with heart disease. *Am. J. Med.*, **77**, 463–70.

132. Metabolic equivalents:

a. True b. False c. True d. True e. False

A metabolic equivalent unit (MET) is used to estimate the metabolic cost of physical activity relative to resting metabolic rate. One metabolic equivalent unit (1 MET) is approximately 3.5 ml of oxygen consumed per kg of body weight per minute. Therefore, 1 MET = the resting metabolic rate. Research has identified the energy requirements of selected activities, and tables exist listing the MET energy requirements of many activities. This method can therefore be used in intensity monitoring, allowing the physician to select an activity which falls within the desired exercise intensity – thereby factoring in the 'desired intensity'. It is particularly helpful in cardiac rehabilitation patients, whose heart rate response may be blunted by cardiac failure or cardiogenic drugs so that heart rate response is not an appropriate way to monitor exercise intensity safely. The MET intensity monitoring system can easily be interchanged with heart rate response intensity monitoring and a Borg scale rating of perceived exertion exercise intensity monitoring. An example of the uses of the metabolic equivalent system follows:

> An individual with a functional capacity of 10 MET (VO_2 max = 35 ml/kg per minute) is advised to take exercise at a level of 40–60 per cent of his functional capacity. Activities such as leisure cycling (3.5 METs), gardening (4.4 METs) and golfing (4.9 METs) can therefore be selected, as they fall within the desired zone of 40–60 per cent of the functional capacity.

Further reading: O'Brien, C. P. (1996). Exercise prescription, lessening the risk of physical activity. *J. Cardiovasc. Risk*, **3**(2), 141–7.

133. Body composition:

a. False b. True c. False d. True e. True

Since ancient times, anthropocentric assessment of the athlete has been part and parcel of the sports person's preparation. Body composition assessment in particular has gained much interest over the last two decades. Research has indicated that aerobic performance is significantly improved by a lowered body fat percentage. Two commonly encountered methods of body composition analysis included body fat percentage analysis and body mass index analysis. Body fat percentage initially involved body weight weighing in and out of water. Presently, however, the most commonly encountered system is to use a four-site calliper reading method. This involves skin fold calliper readings at the anterior superior iliac crest, triceps, biceps and below the spine of the scapula. These four readings (in cm) are added together and applied to body fat percentage tables, which estimates a body fat percentage reading. This is a common component of any physiological assessment or work-up. The body mass index method is more commonly used to assess large populations. This calculation is achieved by dividing the weight in kilograms by the height in metres squared. Normal individuals have a reading of below 25 kg/m^2, obese individuals have a reading greater than 30 kg/m^2 and individuals between

27 kg/m^2 and 30 kg/m^2 are considered to be overweight. Body mass index assessment has now become a common component in all health screening work-ups.

Further reading: Lusaki, H. C. (1987). Methods for assessment of the human body composition: traditional and new. *Am. J. Clin. Nut.* **46**, 537-56.

Therapy and radiology

134. Steroid arthropathy:

a. True b. False c. False d. False e. True

Steroid arthropathy is a well-recognized potential complication of corticosteroid therapy. Many practitioners in the field of musculo-skeletal and sports medicine fear the consequences of steroid injections in an otherwise non-pathological joint. The evidence, however, suggests that it is oral steroids in particular that court the complication of steroid arthropathy, especially when taken in the presence of an associated underlying disease process such as rheumatoid arthritis or chronic alcohol abuse. Systemic disease and chronic alcohol abuse may leave the liver liable to fatty infiltrates and, in the presence of oral steroid therapy, this may result in fatty emboli which can lodge in subchondral bone. This can result in cell death, micro fracture, sequestration and subsequent osteonecrosis. Initial reports of steroid arthropathy were in the late 1950s, and since that time there have only been six cases reported in international literature relating to intra-articular steroids causing joint degeneration. Of these six cases, five had a multiplicity of injections over a 2-year period and four were taking concurrent non-steroidal anti-inflammatories; four also had a systemic disease. It is clear that oral steroids can cause osteonecrosis. The most commonly affected joints are the hip and shoulder. This side effect of oral steroid therapy, however, appears to occur more frequently in the presence of systemic disease and chronic alcohol abuse.

Further reading: Cameron, G. (1995). Steroid arthropathy: myth or reality? A review of the evidence. *J. Orthopaed. Med.*, **17**(2), 12-15.

135. Therapeutic cold laser treatment:

a. False b. True c. False d. False e. False

Lasers are light amplifiers that emit energy in the visible and infrared regions of the electromagnetic spectrum. Lasers emit their energy in pulses, and research has shown that lower dose laser treatment has a positive effect on wound healing and on pain reduction. The laser beam is absorbed by tissues that have a high water content. The actual method of the laser therapeutic effect is not completely understood; however, increased mitochondrial activity, vascularity of wounds and RNA in the endoplasmic reticulum of animals has been reported, as have alterations in the mediators of information.

Further reading: Enwemeka, C. S. (1988). Laser biostimulation of healing wounds: specific effects and mechanism of action. *J. Orthopaed. Sports Phys. Ther.*, **9**(10), 333-338.

136. Injection therapy:

a. False b. True c. True d. True e. True

Soft tissue aspiration and medication injection is useful both as a diagnostic and as a therapeutic tool for musculoskeletal injuries. Aspiration helps relieve pressure and pain by removing blood, pus or inflammatory fluid, and can assist in improving the patient's range of motion and making the soft tissue structure more amenable to rehabilitation. Corticosteroid injection can provided further relief and healing. A variety of musculoskeletal disorders, including impingement syndromes, rotator cuff injuries, epicondylitis, tendon injuries and ganglion disorders, can benefit from aspiration and injection techniques. However, these techniques are absolutely contraindicated if a patient has sepsis or localized cellulitis. Injection therapy is also contraindicated if a patient has a septic arthritis. Relative contraindications for injection include previous site injections of greater than 160 mg of steroid. Previously, it was considered that three or four injections was a rule of thumb; however, as the present recommendations are for significantly lower dose steroid injections (10 mg), a more appropriate approach is to quantify the actual number of milligrams injected at a particular site. Pregnancy is also a relative contraindication, due to the possible effects on the foetus – namely spina bifida. Diabetics must be carefully monitored, as insulin requirements may alter following a corticosteroid injection. Injection therapy should also be avoided following an acute injury because the corticosteroid may alter the collagen formation, resulting in the formation of weaker type 2 collagen. Injecting unco-operative patients should also be avoided, as this may prove too stressful for both patient and doctor; in these cases, iontophoresis is probably a more appropriate therapy.

Further reading: Birrer, R. B. (1992). Aspiration and corticosteroid injections. *Phys. Sports Med.*, **20**(12), 57-71.

137. Shoulder radiology:

a. False b. True c. False d. True e. False

Plain X-rays form an essential part of shoulder examination. Four routine views of the shoulder give adequate information about both soft tissue and bony pathology. AP views in internal and external rotation visualize fractures at the gleno-humeral joint, osteoarthritis at the gleno-humeral and acromioclavicular joints and calcifications of the supraspinatus tendons. An axillary or lateral view can demonstrate Hill–Sachs and bony Bankart lesions, which are seen in patients who have recurring anterior shoulder dislocations. A supraspinatus outlet view should also be taken in cases of suspected rotator cuff injury, as this view allows observation of the shape of the acromion. Three morphological shapes of the acromion have been described: flat, curved and hooked. Rotator cuff injuries are more prevalent in patients who have hooked or curved acromions. Therefore, such a radiological finding can be helpful in equivocal cases of rotator cuff injury. Radiology is also essential to identify primary bone tumours, metastases or Pancoast's tumours, which may mimic a rotator cuff injury.

Further reading: Bigliani, L. Y., Morrison, D. S. and April, E. W. (1986). The morphology of the acromion and its relationship to rotator cuff tears. *Orthopaed. Trans.*, **10**, 228.

Suggested reading

Sports medicine:
Strauss, R. H. (1991). *Sports Medicine*, 2nd edn. W. B. Saunders.

The team physician:
Mellion, M. B., Walsh, W. M. and Shelton, G. L. (1990). *The Team Physician's Handbook*, Mosby Year Book. Hanley and Belfus.

Sports injuries:
Reid, D. C. (1992). *Sports Injury Assessment and Rehabilitation.* Churchill Livingstone.

Musculoskeletal medicine:
Apley, A. G. and Solomon, L. (1994). *Concise System of Orthopaedics and Fractures*, 2nd edn. Butterworth-Heinemann.

Special groups:
Press, J. M. (1993). Physical medicine and rehabilitation. *Sports Med.*, **5(1)**. W. B. Saunders.
Agostini, R. (1994). Clinics. *Sports Med.*, **13(2)**. W. B. Saunders.
Reider, B. (1991). The school-age athlete. *Sports Med.* W. B. Saunders.

Drugs, supplements and toxicology:
Mottram, D. R. (1995). *Drugs in Sport*, 2nd edn. Routledge.
Fuentes, R. J., Rosenberd, J. M. and Davies, A. (1996). *Athletic Drug Reference.* Glaxo Wellcome Inc.

Anatomy:
Kendall, F. P., McCreary, E. K. and Provance, P. (1993). *Muscle Testing and Function,* 4th edn. Lippincott Williams and Wilkins.

Cardiology and sport:
Pollock, M. L. and Schmidt, D. H. (1995). *Heart Disease and Rehabilitation*, 3rd edn. Human Kinetics.

Exercise physiology:
Reilly, T., Secher, N., Snell, P. and Williams, C. (1990). *Physiology of Sports*, 1st edn. E & FN Spon Ltd.
Wilmore, J. H. and Costill, D. L. (1994). *Physiology of Sport and Exercise.* Human Kinetics.

Therapeutics and radiology:
Lennard, T. A. (1995). *Physiatric Procedures in Clinical Practice.* Hanley and Belfus Inc.
Bowerman, J. W. (1977). *Radiology and Injury in Sport.* Appleton-Century-Crofts.
Bloem, J. L. and Sartoris, D. J. (1992). *MRI and CT of the Musculoskeletal System, A Text Atlas.* Lippincott Williams and Wilkins.
Van Holsbeeck, M. and Introcaso, J. A. (1999). *Musculoskeletal Ultrasound*, 2nd edn. Mosby.

Index

Index entries refer to Question/ Answer numbers

9 780750 629492

Printed and bound by CPI Group (UK) Ltd, Croydon, CR0 4YY

03/10/2024

01040848-0009